Whole Food Nutrition:
The Missing Link in
Vitamin Therapy

Whole Food Nutrition: The Missing Link in Vitamin Therapy

The Difference Between Nutrients WITHIN
Foods vs. Isolated Vitamins &
How They Affect Your Health

Vic Shayne, Ph.D.

iUniverse.com, Inc.
San Jose New York Lincoln Shanghai

Whole Food Nutrition: The Missing Link in Vitamin Therapy
The Difference Between Nutrients WITHIN Foods vs.
Isolated Vitamins & how they affect your health

Published by iUniverse.com, Inc.

For information address:
iUniverse.com, Inc.
5220 S 16th, Ste. 200
Lincoln, NE 68512
www.iuniverse.com

ISBN: 0-595-14476-4

Printed in the United States of America

DEDICATION

This book is dedicated to future generations who must understand that we are all a part of Nature, and to destroy Nature is to destroy humanity. The food, air, water and harmony of nature that sustains us all must be safeguarded from profiteers who continually threaten to undermine the balance of our fragile ecology by means of alteration, destruction and deceit. The truth is that we need real, whole and complex foods to survive in health and happiness.

EPIGRAPH

Whole foods contain a complex, interwoven network of interrelated nutrients needed for biochemical function and cellular health, repair and vitality. Whole foods contain vitamins, minerals, amino acids and countless other nutrients balanced by the innate intelligence of Nature. Vitamin pills, on the other hand, NEVER contain the rest of the whole food complex. Once removed from their original food complexes, vitamins are not nutrients, but rather chemicals. This is the scientific and clinical argument for the use of whole food concentrate supplements.

CONTENTS

ACKNOWLEDGEMENTS

Special thanks to Janice Shayne, CHt, president of NutriPlex Formulas, Inc., for choosing to educate and inform doctors and their patients worldwide about the benefits, uses and uniqueness of whole food supplementation for health and repair. Thanks also to my mentors, Dr. Richard P. Murray and Dr. Gilbert D. Williams, for selflessly sharing their experiences and expertise in natural healthcare, biochemistry and biology. And special thanks to author/researcher/herbalist James Duke, Ph.D. and Leslie Taylor, N.D. for answering my inquiries on my never-ending search for natural solutions to health concerns. I also appreciate the friendship and clinical feedback received from Dr. Russell Shurtleff. And thanks to my Qi Gong teachers, Andrew Chung and Zhu Xilin.

WHOLE FOOD NUTRITION VS. SYNTHETIC SUPPLEMENTATION

Whole foods, found in their natural, undisturbed, unprocessed state, contain a host of interactive nutrients too numerous to categorize. Some of these nutrients are vitamins, others are minerals. And there's much more. Once scientists isolated vitamins, minerals, amino acids and enzymes in a laboratory, they were able to test their functions and efficacy against disease and symptomatology. Yet somewhere along the way, modern science and marketing have allowed (persuaded?) us to forget that nutrients NEVER exist in isolation in their natural states. There can be no argument that isolated and synthetic vitamins produce pharmacological effects which show promise against disease symptoms. However, for any doctor or patient seeking a truly natural approach to healthcare, we must consider the synergistic effects of nutrients contained in their natural, whole states before deciding how, when and why to use supplementation. The human body and its environment is so extremely complex and dynamic, that many practitioners, including myself, would rather surrender to the innate intelligence of nature than to presume that it is even possible to achieve wholistic results with isolated, chemical supplements. Therefore, this book is not an argument pitting whole foods against isolates, but rather a study in exploring the cofactors and constituents in whole foods that are absent—but still needed by the body's biochemistry—in isolated, synthetic supplements.

Some researchers feel that supplementation with isolated substances such as vitamins, minerals and amino acids runs the risk of creating a chain reaction in the human physiology. This is a very real possibility, given today's zeal for fad supplements, megadosing, supplement abuses, self-diagnosis, and self-prescribing. For instance, the layman who reads that niacin is an important B vitamin that everyone needs, is really getting just a part of the whole picture. Left out is the important consideration that the rest of the other B vitamins as well as their cofactors are needed. This same person may next read that tryptophan is important for synthesizing niacin; so he then runs out for tryptophan supplements. There is no end to this chase. In another scenario, an athlete may "discover" the need for zinc which he then supplements by the handful only to accidentally impair his supply of vitamin A, vitamin C, hormones, iron and copper. Copper deficiency, in turn, can increase blood cholesterol. From here, many physiological systems may be altered, interrupted or damaged, including the adrenal glands, endocrine system, prostate health, brain chemical balance, blood cells and cardiovascular system, to name only a few, as each nutrient is linked to another in an infinite and wondrous system.

In another example of creating imbalances within the body's delicate biochemical system, an overdose of vitamin E may cause bleeding as in vitamin K deficiency.[1] Vitamin D excess (doses 2-3 times the Recommended Daily Allowance) can be toxic when it leads to high blood calcium levels and calcification of soft tissue. "Moderately high consumption [of vitamin D] over a long period of time may increase the risk of atherosclerosis."[2] Vitamin A toxicity is a concern with synthetic forms of vitamin A, especially in pregnancy, where it may potentially lead to birth defects. Yet, vitamin A as a natural, food constituent is very important in the diet of pregnant mothers.

---

[1] Ronzio, Ph.D., Robert, *The Encyclopedia of Nutrition and Good Health*, Facts on File, Inc., New York, 1997, page 451.

[2] Ronzio, page 449, re: Fraser, D.R., "Vitamin D," *Lancet*, 345 (January 14, 1995), pages 104-107.

Manganese overdose may interfere with iron absorption. And excessive calcium intake may interfere with manganese. Large doses of potassium can lead to electrolyte imbalances, especially for those with kidney disease, diabetes or heart problems. A complete description of how isolated vitamins and minerals are dependent and interrelated is seemingly impossible to calculate due to the variables both known and unknown.

Not only do vitamins and minerals exist as parts of delicately balanced cofactors and constituents found in whole foods, but so do amino acids (the building blocks of proteins). It is common today, especially among athletes (professional and amateur), to ingest large amounts of isolated amino acids in an attempt to build and repair muscle that is damaged in the catabolism that takes place with exertion, injury, vigorous exercise and strenuous activity. Amino acid researchers Eric Braverman, M.D. and Carl Pfeiffer, M.D. caution: "Because many of the amino acids are absorbed and metabolized in a similar fashion, there is a great deal of competition between molecules. Sometimes, one amino acid can cancel the effect of others. This adds to the overall complexity of prescribing amino acids to treat disease. For example, amino acids compete for absorption with others in the same group, e.g., the aromatic amino acid group (tryptophan, tyrosine and phenylalanine) and can inhibit one another's passage into the brain."[3] To study the complex world of amino acids and their interactions, relationships and synergists, the reader is invited to study Dr. Braverman's, *The Healing Nutrients Within: Facts, Findings and New Research on Amino Acids* (Keats Publishing, 1987).

Modern medicine has been blamed with an astounding incidence rate of iatrogenic (resultant from modern medical treatment) illness, but in all fairness, this author would suspect that so-called "alternative healthcare treatment" leads to side effects, illness and symptomatology by the thou-

---

[3] Braverman, M.D., Eric R. and Carl C. Pfeiffer, M.D., Ph.D., *The Healing Nutrients Within, Facts, findings and New Research on Amino Acids*, Keats Publishing, New Canaan, Connecticut, 1987, pages 14-15.

sands. But the latter cases are most likely to go unnoticed by the medical community because inappropriate supplementation creates effects that are as varied and complex as any one of the billions of human individuals inhabiting our complex and dynamic planet This is the greatest argument for leaving nutrient dosages, vitamins, minerals, amino acids, and enzymes to the balance of nature as found in whole, natural, pure foods.

THE INNATE INTELLIGENCE OF NATURE: IDENTIFYING THE PARTS & APPRECIATING THE WHOLE

In the short history of humankind, we have risen rapidly to scientific heights by the powers of insight, imagination, willpower, trial and error, and sheer accident. As a result, we have achieved wonders in understanding the mechanisms of our bodies and our environment. Yet, in science's attempt to recreate life itself, we are no closer to the feat than we were at the dawn of time. For all of our understanding about life—cells, microbes, bacteria, genetics and nerve impulses—we still cannot create life out of lifeless matter. The mysteries of what makes one organism alive versus non-living remains a transcendental aspect of our existence that perhaps will never be ascertained. Although we can, through scientific observation, identify why something is said to be alive, we are confounded as to how to bring a non-living entity to life, despite our intimate understanding of its physiology, biology, physics, anatomy, psychology and energy. At this juncture, it seems, the spiritual aspect of life is forever set apart from our scientific ability and know-how. For all of our technological and scientific genius, the best we can come up with is the saying "Only God can make a tree." Whether we view God as a real entity or a metaphor for the transcendent mystery of life is immaterial and best left up to one's religious persuasion. But for the purposes of this study on whole food nutrition, it suffices to say that scientists have yet to recreate (or even come close to recreating) a real, living food due to its complexity and energetic constituents.

Nature appears to have an innate intelligence. All things natural, including humans, animals, plants and even the cycles of life—weather, planetary orchestration and motion, the ebb and flow of the ocean, etc.—are complex in their existence. This means that natural entities are made up of a series of co-dependent parts that cannot work on their own; nor do they exist by themselves, despite how valuable they are. A leaf does not appear without the rest of the plant; a brain does not exist without a body; a cloud does not exist without a sky; a feather cannot take flight without a bird; and a real vitamin does not exist unless it is contained in a food. In nature, we find whole entities in unique and awesome systems. The inter workings of infinite (measurable and unmeasurable; tangible and energetic) parts contribute to making a successful and living whole. Further, these parts are kept in a natural balance for optimum function, performance, protection, recreation and movement. To remain in balance, the entire entity depends upon its environment—a larger, natural system. For instance, a beautiful bird, no matter how well designed and healthy, cannot live unless it is supported by its environment with food, water, the right temperature, etc. One ecosystem is contained within another, within another, right down to the cell and even further. This is the interdependence of life.

In speaking of nutrition, we are relating to plants and animals as a means of sustenance. Our human bodies are dependent on foods to carry on our varied functions from cells to muscles. Internally, we need foods and the nutrients contained within them for the health of our pumping hearts and thinking brains; our bending joints and our powerful muscles; our breathing lungs and our chewing jaws. Externally, we need food nutrients to carry on many tasks—typing at the computer, solving problems, planting trees, harvesting crops, driving to work, cleaning our houses, jogging around the block, and even completing the circle/cycle by preserving our environment so that these functions will continue to be possible. We are as much dependent upon our environment as our environment is dependent upon us, for we are a part of the "complex" that sustains us as life forms. The Native Americans understood this as well as any culture. When the white civilization destroyed their buffalo near the end of the 19th century, the Natives understood that this was the beginning of the end of their life cycle. They understood and accurately predicted the toll that abuse of the environment would take on civilization. They knew that nature sustains man and animal alike, and to think oneself above nature was the beginning of the end. Now, more than a hundred years later, we are just beginning to understand the enormity of our responsibility to be as much a part of nature as a contributor to its perpetuation.

Nature has long fascinated and perplexed humankind. This is why we like to take things apart to see how they work. Such a task is easier accomplished with an unnatural contraption such as a clock full of springs, gears and pins. Yet with living objects, it is a bit more difficult to understand how things work, because once apart, they cease to retain their intimate relationships, bonds and interchanges. Creating or recreating life from dead, isolated parts remains in the sphere of science fiction as in the Frankenstein monster. Regardless, most of today's scientific body of knowledge is related to the study of things *out of* their natural environments and separated from their synergists and cofactors. Unfortunately, to study some things means to kill them, destroy them and fractionate them (look at them in isolation apart from the rest of the being). In this seemingly illogical way, scientists try to figure out why specific nutrients work; or, what it is in a specific food that creates a specific action upon our cells. Scientists want to know how a particular vitamin or mineral affects our bodies via molecular exchange. Although scientists may know that vitamin E is good for our hearts, this is not sufficient knowledge. Researchers also want to know HOW vitamin E leads to better health—how it affects cellular function; how it interacts with other food constituents, its antioxidant capabilities, etc. This is a noble investigation—looking for solutions to problems. But the solutions may lead to more problems.

Where then does science go wrong? Once scientists identify which vitamin in a particular food affects a specific bodily function, instead of appreciating that the vitamin is part of an integral, complex system which is inseparable from the rest of the nutrients in the whole food, there is a tendency to believe that the isolated substance (a vitamin, in this example) works the same exact way when no longer a part of the whole food complex. In analogy, we can say that although we know and understand that fingers are the body parts used for typing a letter, we fully understand that without the rest of the body, including the brain, arms, wrist, nerves, muscles, tendons, etc., the fingers cannot by themselves naturally type a letter, or even of their own volition make their way to the computer for that matter. Similarly, naturalists argue that a vitamin which is no longer contained within a whole food cannot really act as a vitamin at all, but rather only as some drug-like substance. In this case, the vitamin is no longer part of a living substance (a real food), but is instead converted into a chemical, as opposed to a *bio*chemical. (*bio*=living+chemical).

Among the "experts" exists a fundamental difference of opinion—that of the naturalist versus that of the chemist.

In the end we must ask ourselves: if vitamins and minerals and other food components can be duplicated or isolated, why do we need to eat foods at all? The answer is simple: because foods are complex, living substances containing parts and components that we have yet to duplicate or arrange according to the innate intelligence of nature. As scientists, we can attempt to copy (albeit imperfectly) parts of nature, but we cannot make life from the nonliving; nor can we duplicate the intricacies and relationships of the whole food complex.

In his extensive research and cultivation of cereal grasses, Ronald Seibold, MS, has discovered:

> Through the 1940s and 1950s, cereal grasses were found to contain a number of 'factors' which had different health-related effects on animals. In addition to the growth and fertility factors, grass was shown to contain factors which support the growth of lactobacilli and other beneficial intestinal bacteria.

Cereal grasses contain a factor which blocks the development of scurvy (vitamin C deficiency) which follows the feeding of glucoascorbic acid. This effect could not be duplicated by the feeding of vitamin C (ascorbic acid). Other reports describe a cereal grass factor which blocks the formation of histamine-induced ulcers in guinea pigs. Clinical studies conducted by Dr. Cheney at Stanford in 1950 demonstrated that green vegetables contain a factor which promotes the healing of peptic ulcers.

By 1950, all the nutrients now considered essential to the human diet (with the exception of selenium) had been identified. But researchers continued to describe green food 'factors' which could not be correlated with any known nutrient. In 1957, Ershoff again demonstrated the growth stimulating effect of a green food factor for guinea pigs. All cereal grasses produced similar results...

In 1960, the same laboratory described a water-soluble factor in alfalfa which improved utilization of vitamin A in rats. This factor was shown to be distinct from known nutrients, including the carotenes. In 1966, Dr. George Briggs and others identified a 'plant factor' in grasses, alfalfa and broccoli, which...provided significant growth stimulation when fed to guinea pigs...To this day the 'Grass Juice Factor' in young green plants, required for life and health in guinea pigs, has still not been identified as any of the known nutrients.[4]

[4] Seibold, MS, Ronald L., *Cereal Grass, What's in it for you!*, Wilderness Community Education Foundation, Kansas, 1990, pages 24-25, citing: Colio, L and Babb, V, 1948. Study of a new stimulatory growth factor, *Journal of Biological Chemistry*, 174: 405-409; Cheney, G, 1950. Anti-peptic ulcer dietary factor. *Journal of the American Dietetic Association*, 26:668-672.; Woolley, D and Krampitz, L, 1943. Production of a scurvy-like condition by feeding of a compound structurally related to ascorbic acid. *Journal of Experimental Medicine*, 78:333; Kohler, G 1953. The unidentified vitamins of grass and alfalfa. *Feedstuffs*,

This small bit of information regarding "unknown" factors in foods should tell us two things: First, we must be careful not to be so conceited as to think that our science has outsmarted and surpassed the ancient wisdom of Mother Nature; and second, that we must recognize that the unknown may be as much of the secret to life and vitality as the known.

Vitamins and minerals and other food constituents are part of a greater whole. As we shall see, not only do vitamins need other cofactors to work, but they also need subfactors. For example, vitamin A needs fat-splitting enzymes, minerals, amino acids and other vitamins for optimum benefit and assimilation. But vitamin A also needs all of its subfactors—not just beta carotene, but also delta carotene, retinal, retinol, and retinoic acid. Similarly, vitamin D and calcium work together. Calcium balances sodium and phosphorus. Vitamin E and selenium are synergists. Vitamin E acts as a cofactor in oxidative phosphorylation reactions; while vitamin C protects vitamin E from oxidation. Riboflavin is a cofactor of thiamin. Choline depends upon folic acid to transfer methyl groups; and choline depends on vitamin B_{12} for its synthesis. The inter workings of vitamins, minerals, amino acids, essential fatty acids, enzymes, coenzymes and other substances are immeasurable. The balance of nutrients is inherent in nature's live foods and is admittedly beyond the full comprehension of man and his limited science.

Can we say, then, that fractionated or synthetic vitamins do not work? To answer this question, we must define the word "work." Yes, they work, but as drug-like, or pharmacological, substances, not as food nutrients. Certainly, out of their food complexes they are no longer part of a living

---

August 8, 1953; Erschoff, B, 1957. Beneficial effects of alfalfa and other succulent plants on the growth of immature guinea pigs fed a mineralized dried milk ration. *Journal of Nutrition*, 62- 62:295-312.; Erschoff, B and Hernandez, H, 1960. An unidentified water-soluble factor in alfalfa which improves utilization of vitamin A. *Journal of Nutrition*, 70:313-320; Lakhanpal, R, Davis, J, Typpo, J and Briggs, G, 1966. Evidence for an unidentified growth factor from alfalfa and other plant sources for young guinea pigs. *Journal of Nutrition*, 89:341-346.

unit and are devoid of their cofactors and subfactors. Isolated vitamins may eradicate symptoms or *seem* to cure diseases, but they are not nutrients and do not feed the cells with live constituents created by nature to sustain life and support biochemistry. Due to the complexity of the human biochemistry and physiology, evidence shows that isolated "nutrients" (i.e., chemicals) often seem to resolve symptoms, yet they concomitantly create new ones. Because vitamins, minerals and amino acids require cofactors to work, by feeding the body isolated substances, the body is forced to surrender its own stores of cofactors. The net effect is "borrowing from Peter to pay Paul," potentially setting off a chain reaction (previously illustrated) of biochemical imbalances, many of which may not be immediately apparent as symptoms or illness. As we shall see, the human biochemistry, as a microcosm of nature itself, is far too complex and dynamic to predict the adverse effects of ingesting isolated substances, whether so-called natural, or synthetic.

Whole Food Nutrients: Too Complex to Identify

"Vitamin and mineral supplement sales are a $6.4 billion market; herbal supplements bring in at least $1.2 billion. The most dramatic increase in sales has occurred in the use of single vitamin supplements such as vitamin C, E, calcium and antioxidant tablets. The FDA reports that 53 percent of adults, or 101 million Americans, take nutritional supplements, with about 58 percent of women and 47 percent of men using vitamins or minerals. Typical users have some college education and fall in the middle to upper income range."[5]

There you have it—intelligent people, in the millions, are taking substances which defy the logic of nature and biochemistry. Although the action is well-intended, to many biochemical researchers, it is misguided and resultant from powerful marketing stimuli, misinformation, high expectations, unsubstantiated anecdotal claims and partial truths. Vitamin supplements are as far from being foods as are drugs. Some would even argue that they are one and the same thing—both being lifeless compounds able to affect (stimulate and suppress) bodily functions. As we shall see, food substances, including vitamins, are extremely complex and never exist alone in nature; they need synergists and the right environment to

[5] *Journal of the American Medical Association*, April 10, 1996, as reviewed in the Food Safety Notebook, April 1996; and Pulse, (American Dietetic Association) Fall 1996. *Networking News*, (American Dietetic Association) Winter 1997.

function. They need to be part of a live (live enzyme-containing) whole food to be naturally balanced and functional.

Most nutrition textbooks concur: "In general, nutrients are absorbed best from foods, in which they are dispersed among other ingredients that may facilitate their absorption. Taken in pure, concentrated form, they are more likely to interfere with each other's absorption or with the absorption of the nutrients in foods eaten at the same time. Minerals provide examples: zinc hinders copper and calcium absorption, iron hinders zinc absorption, calcium hinders magnesium and iron absorption, and magnesium hinders the absorption of calcium and iron. The same interference takes place when people use foods that are fortified with added minerals, another reason to rely on ordinary whole foods for optimal absorption of nutrients."[6]

When isolating a specific vitamin or mineral, or in creating a synthetic vitamin, some of the most important factors in food nutrition are disregarded, ignored or overlooked. In particular are factors known as *phytochemicals*, very often the "missing link" in the curative effect of isolated/synthetic supplements.

Getting All The Vitamins & Minerals You Need From Your Diet—An Oversimplification

Older textbooks on nutrition, as well as standard the advice of the allopathic, modern medical community, used to be to avoid supplements altogether because "you can get all of the vitamins and minerals you need from the foods in your diet." Dietitians showed us how to do it as they carefully plotted out the ideal diet in an oversimplified, off-target diagram called the Food Pyramid, which as of this writing, is still going strong and being taught to school children across the nation.

---

[6] Hamilton, Eva May Nunnelley, Eleanor Noss Whitney, Frances Sienkiewicz Sizer, *Nutrition: Concepts and Controversies* West Publishing Company, St. Paul, MN, 1991, page 234-235.

Can we get all the minerals and vitamins we need from our diet? This is a loaded question. First, people in modern societies do not have ideal diets and very few understand or care to implement a good diet. The drive to eat tasty foods and convenient foods far outweighs the drive to create and maintain health through foods. This is especially true in the face of our quick-fix attitude toward EVERYTHING. We are constantly being bombarded with marketing messages assuring us that a cure comes to us in the form of a pill, injection or surgical procedure. It is not in our social heritage to grasp the true meaning of food as "nature's medicine." Perhaps the traditional Chinese, who discovered the wisdom of implementing food cures thousands of years ago, may embrace the idea of eating for better health. But to the Western world, this idea is as foreign as walking in nature as a means of therapy.

Today's modern diet is deplorable, despite that special interest groups such as sugar growers, food irradiators, genetic engineering corporations, fast food restaurateurs and the dairy industry are trying to convince us otherwise. The modern diet is replete with chemicals, toxins, industrial wastes and altered foods never meant for human (or animal) consumption. These substances are unfit for meeting the needs of biochemical and physiological processes. Even worse, not only do today's so-called foods not supply essential nutrients, but they also create disease with ingredients such as refined sugar, refined grains, synthetic vitamins (enriched and fortified), artificial sweeteners, chemical excipients, artificial flavorings, pesticide residues, synthetic chemical fertilizers, preservatives, emulsifiers and so forth. Even good, whole foods may be rendered nearly useless, or perhaps harmful, merely by cooking. Vitamin C, for instance, is known to be easily destroyed upon exposure to air or in cooking. Amino acids and essential fatty acids are destroyed or chemically altered when cooked. The difference between a good food and a bad one may only be in the preparation for mealtime. Barbecues, microwave ovens, aluminum cooking pans, fluoridated water[7] and cauldrons often are involved in promoting disease as much as the non-foods themselves.

Even if one were to have a "really good" diet, we cannot ignore the nutrient-depleting lifestyle that is most common here in the 21st century. We are the effects of stress (mental, emotional and physical), pollution, depression, high blood pressure, allergies, mood swings, genetics, vaccinations and so much more that diet alone cannot handle.

The modern diet fails to meet the needs of the human organism, leading more than one thinker to opine, "America may be the MOST FED nation on earth, but certainly not the BEST FED." Hence the need for supplementation: The alternative to the typical isolated/fractionated supplements is with *whole food concentrates* in which whole foods have been concentrated into tablet/capsule form without destroying enzymes and by keeping intact the original food complex.

One of the biggest problems any natural healthcare doctor has in getting his/her patient well is patient compliance and cooperation. Only in theory can we get all the minerals and vitamins we need from our diet. Even if one was to adopt a healthy, nutrient-dense diet from this day forward, we still must address the [dietary] "sins of the past." In other words, we must be concerned with nutrient deficiencies which exist now and may have taken many years to create. Perhaps there are even genetic or traumatic (accidents, iatrogenic illness, chemical poisoning, etc.) influences upon our physiology that demand extra attention. In this regard, supplementation is

---

7 Preventive Dental Health Assn: "The Dangers of Fluoridation & Alternatives to Fluoride; Elke Babluk—Fluoride: Protected Pollutant or Panacea?, 1999; *Scholarly Journal of the International Society for Fluoride Research*, on the web: www.fluoride-journal.com; Val Verlerian, Fluorides & Fluoridation, Leading Edge Research Group, on the web: trufax.or/fluoride/fluorides.html, 1999; Schacter, M.D., Michael, "The Dangers of Fluoride & Fluoridation, on the web at www.healthy.net, 1999; Taylou, DDS, Joyal, "Fluoride: Dentistry's Boondoggle, on the web at healthynet/dentistry, 2000.

recommended. In looking at vitamin C alone, for instance, nutritional researcher Elson Haas, M.D., writes, "Vitamin C is used up even more rapidly under stressful conditions, with alcohol use, and with smoking. Vitamin C blood levels of smokers are much lower than those of nonsmokers given the same intakes. Other situations and substances that reduce absorption or increase utilization include fever, viral illness, antibiotics, cortisone, aspirin and other pain medicines, environmental toxins such as DDT, petroleum products, or carbon monoxide, and exposure to heavy metals such as lead, mercury, or cadmium. Sulfa antibiotics increase elimination of vitamin C from the body by two to three times."[8] By merely being a member of modern society, each of us faces vitamin deficiency owing to myriad causes.

WHOLE FOOD SUPPLEMENTS

To meet the needs of nutrient deficiencies as well as the nutrient depleters we face each day, whole food concentrate supplements may be the best answer. These are the only types of supplements that closest achieve harmony with the biochemistry. Whole food supplements are made of foods (to be discussed in more detail later in this book) instead of chemicals or fractionated (isolated) vitamins, minerals or other parts of foods. Not as beneficial as fresh foods off the farm, whole food concentrate supplements are the next best means of meeting the nutrient requirements of the body's biochemical and physiological systems. Whole food concentrate supplements are whole, real and natural foods that have been concentrated into tablet, powder or capsule form to be used in conjunction with a wise and sound diet and lifestyle.

---

[8] Haas, M.D., Elson, *Staying Healthy With Nutrition*, 1999.

More About Food Nutrients

With all of the billions of dollars spent on vitamins and drugs, still no one is arguing that we can do without good old-fashioned food. Ironically, however, it can be argued that the modern diet does not even consist mostly of real food, but rather processed, refined, overcooked, pasteurized, devitalized and chemicalized concoctions appealing to the taste buds and senses of smell, touch and sight rather than the biochemical needs of the body. Like vitamin supplements, such "food" is absent of enzymes and is essentially dead; without enzymatic activity. Real food remains our only hope for nutrient intake and assimilation in this day and age of fast food, instant food, enriched and fortified foods and foods that are more chemicals than nutrients.

Foods (pure and whole) are our best sources of vitamins, minerals, enzymes, proteins, amino acids, trace minerals, essential fatty acids, and phytochemicals (also called phytonutrients).

Efficacy of Foods; Food Studies

Most studies regarding vitamins and minerals are on isolated substances. Whole food studies yield health-promoting facts, yet no singular substance may take credit for the overall efficacy of the food. Whole food diets (particularly those rich in natural fruits and vegetables) point to healthier people not only because they contain vitamins or groups of vitamins, *but rather because they contain all of their natural synergists in an interwoven and balanced form that the body recognizes in the overall physiological picture.* In one study, for example, a diet of fruits and vegetables was found to result in a lowered risk of stroke. *The Journal of the American Medical Association* showed that those who eat at least five servings of fruit and vegetables a day have a 31 percent lower risk of stroke than those who eat less than three servings. It may be concluded, by logical extension, that by eating such amounts of fruits and vegetables (five servings), there is little time and room left for consumption of some of the more harmful types of foodstuffs. Or perhaps health benefits point to enzyme-rich, unprocessed foods containing real, natural and whole sources of vitamins, minerals, etc.[9]

"Researchers from the Harvard School of Public Health in Boston studied the link between daily fruit and vegetable intake and ischemic stroke in 75,596 women between the ages of 34 to 59 enrolled in the Nurses' Health Study and followed [these subjects] for 14 years. They also studied these links in 38,683 men between the ages of 40 to 75 who were involved in the Health Professionals' Follow-Up Study, which lasted eight years. None of the participants had cardiovascular disease, cancer, or diabetes at the beginning of the studies. The results showed that the risk of ischemic stroke was 31 percent lower in women who consumed an average of 5.8 servings of fruits and vegetables per day, and in men who consumed an average of 5.1 servings per day, than it was in women or men who consumed less than three servings of fruit and vegetables per day. The lowest risk of ischemic stroke overall was found in men and women who ate the most of certain types of vegetables including broccoli, cabbage, cauliflower and Brussels sprouts, as well as green leafy vegetables, citrus fruits and vitamin C-rich fruits and vegetables. The results also showed that for each increase in the number of servings of fruits and vegetables a day, the risk of ischemic stroke in men and women dropped by a combined average of six percent."[10]

Conversely, in a study sponsored by Harvard Researchers, published in the *Annals of Internal Medicine*, 1999, research shows that a high intake of vitamin C and vitamin E supplements failed to reduce the risk of stroke. Here, researchers compared the eight-year history of antioxidant consumption in 44,000 male health professionals aged 40 to 75.[11]

---

9 *Vitamin News* for October 1999: *Journal of the American Medical Association*

10 *Vitamin News* for October 1999: *Journal of the American Medical Association*, 1999; 282: 1233-1239.

11 *Vitamin News* for October 1999: *Annals of Internal Medicine 1999; 130-963-970.*

In a study published in the *Journal of Clinical Epidemiology,* 1999, researchers from the University of Cambridge found that people who ate salad and raw vegetables frequently, on a year-round basis, had more than an 80 percent lower risk of type 2 diabetes than people who ate vegetables less often. This study included 1,122 persons between ages 40 and 64.[12]

Research results appearing in the *American Journal of Public Health* showed that whole grain foods reduce the risk of chronic illnesses, according to an Iowa Women's Health Study. Researchers assessed the whole grain intake in more than 38,000 women. "During the nine years of follow-up, the women in the study who reported eating at least one serving per day of whole grain foods had a lower risk of dying of cancer, cardiovascular disease and other disorders than women who ate no whole grain products."[13]

Likewise, results from the Nurses Health Study suggest that women eating two to three servings of whole grains per day in foods such as whole wheat bread, oatmeal or even popcorn reduce the risk of heart disease by nearly 30 percent. More than 75,000 women ages 38-63 were involved in this study.[14]

In one Harvard cancer study, cabbage and broccoli appeared to have reduced the risk of bladder cancer in 47,000 male subjects of the Health Professionals Follow-up Study.[15]

Yet another study showed the efficacy of walnuts in lowering the risk of heart disease. *Preventive Medicine* reported the results of a study of 793 people ages 18-65 who live in a walnut-producing area in France. French researchers claim that "a diet high in walnuts has beneficial effects on blood cholesterol levels and can reduce the risk of heart disease." Those who reported frequently consuming walnut oil and walnuts had higher levels of eneficial HDL cholesterol. The more oil the subjects ate, the greater the benefits, according to researchers.[16]

---

12 Vitamin News for October 1999: *Journal of Clinical Epidemiology,* 1999; 52:329-335.

13 *American Journal of Public Health* 1999; 89: 322-329

14 *American Journal of Clinical Nutrition* 1999; 70: 412-419

15 *Journal of the National Cancer Institute* 1999; 91: 605-613

16 *Preventive Medicine* 1999; 28: 333-339

Phytochemicals & Phytonutrients

Relatively new to the nutritional lexicon is the term *phytochemical*—a term not to be found in the older texts on biochemistry, botany or herbology. By virtue of the mere use of this term, scientists understand that there is much more to food nutrients than just isolated vitamins or minerals. Although there are a wide range of chemicals found in foods—some beneficial and some harmful—the term "phytonutrient" is actually more user-friendly because it refers to the beneficial constituents of foods. However, there's no stopping the misuse of any term, and so phytochemicals and phytonutrients are words used interchangeably.

The American Society of Nutritional Sciences tells us that "phytochemicals have multiple functions. Some attract insects to encourage fertilization while others provide defenses against predators such as viruses and animals. Phytochemicals exhibit diversified physiologic and pharmacologic effects. Active derivatives extracted from leaves, stems, roots, flowers and fruits of plants may be classified into three main categories. The first are compounds such as pyrrolizidine alkaloids, nicotine and hydrazine derivatives that are highly toxic and have no discernible therapeutic use. The second are morphine, digitalis and vinca alkaloids. These may be toxic but can elicit useful physiologic responses for treatment of disease when used in controlled amounts or for defined clinical conditions. The third group may exhibit chemopreventive activity against diseases such as atherosclerosis, cancer and diverticular disease. Most active are high molecular weight fibers (celluloids, pectins, lignins) and low molecular weight compounds (carotenoids, dithiolthiones, flavonoids, indole carbinols, isothiocyanates, mono-and triterpenoids, and thioallyl derivatives)."[17]

---

[17] American Academy of Nutritional Sciences; Goldberg, I., ed. (1994) In: *Functional Foods. Designer Foods, Pharmafoods, Nutraceuticals.* Chapman & Hall, New York, NY ; and Moon, T.E. & Micozzi, M.S., eds. (1989) *Nutrition and Cancer Prevention. Investigating the Role of Micronutrients.* Marcel Dekker, Inc., New York, NY.

"Clinical and laboratory studies currently focus on cardiovascular protection and anticarcinogenic effects of phytochemicals. Risk factors of cardiovascular disease may be ameliorated by lowering cholesterol formation, blocking platelet aggregation, and/or altering prostaglandin formation. Anticancer activities include enhancing detoxification enzymes and antioxidant capacity, inhibition of DNA adduct formation, altering hormone metabolism, and modifying promotion and mechanisms of progression."[18]

Phytochemicals are found in a wide variety of food sources, ranging from cruciferous plants to legumes, and from citrus fruits to roots. Although scientists readily admit that they are uncertain of the quantities of phytochemicals needed in the diet, they are willing to state that the absence of phytochemicals contributes to disease such as cancer and genetic abnormalities. Further, it appears that an excess or imbalance of phytochemicals may create toxic effects. "Most phytochemicals are non-nutritive substances that can be beneficial and/or physiologically or pharmacologically active. Depending on the quantities consumed, duration of consumption, and the conditions of use, most phytochemicals have the potential capacity to produce cellular or tissue injury."[19]

According to the *Journal of the American Dietetic Association,* "Health benefits of these foods [phytochemicals] are best obtained through the consumption of a varied diet using our normal food supply. These phytochemicals and/or health-preserving elements are present in a number of frequently consumed foods, especially fruits, vegetables, grains, legumes, and seeds, and in a number of less frequently consumed foods such as licorice, soy, and green tea. Phytochemicals and food components have been associated with the prevention and/or treatment of at least four of the leading causes of death in this country—cancer, diabetes, cardiovascular disease, and hypertension—and with the prevention and/or treatment

---

[18] ibid.
[19] ibid.

of other medical ailments including neural tube defects, osteoporosis, abnormal bowel function, and arthritis. The National Cancer Institute estimates that one in three cancer deaths are diet related and that 8 of 10 cancers have a nutrition/diet component."[20]

Plant researcher/author James Duke, Ph.D. tells us that plant food and herbs provide nutrients that "are essential to life. Research has now shown that many of us are deficient in several nutrients essential to optimal health, if not essential to life itself. Many of these important, natural ingredients are found in herbs, but not in synthetic pharmaceuticals.

"When synthetic drugs are made from plants, we tend to isolate one or another chemical and throw away the rest of the plant and its medicinal potential. The fava bean, for instance, contains ingredients that could be extracted and used as 'magic-bullet' pharmaceuticals—such as L-dopa, which is used in the treatment of Parkinson's Disease…But why throw away the rest of the bean to make a proprietary monochemical medicine that can be patented by a pharmaceutical company? We should, instead, be studying the synergistic energies of all those phytochemicals and discovering how they work so well together. Those are the studies that will lead us to a true understanding of the many healing qualities of medicinal plants."[21]

Phytochemicals, including known and unknown constituents of plants, are parts of foods that perhaps should be called phyto-*bio*-chemicals because they are live, life-supporting substances. Phytochemicals include vitamins as well as other substances, including flavonoids (of which there are thousands of types), phytoesterols, carotenoids, indoles, comarins, organosulfur compounds, terpenes, saponins, lignans and isothiocyanates.

"Cruciferous plants, such as cabbage and broccoli, are excellent sources of indoles, dithiolthiones, isothiocyanates and chlorophyllins. Legumes (soybeans, peanuts, beans and peas) contain flavonoids, isoflavanoids and

---

[20] *J Am Diet Assoc* 1995;95:493.

[21] Duke, Ph.D., James, *The Green Pharmacy*, Rodale Press, Pennsylvania, 1997.

other polyphenols that act as antioxidants and estrogenic agonists/antagonists. Citrus fruits and licorice root contain mono-and tri-terpenes that act as antioxidants, cholesterol synthesis inhibitors, and stifle growth of rapidly dividing cells. Thioallyl derivatives are found in garlic, leeks and onion, and prevent thrombi formation, decrease cholesterol synthesis, and prevent DNA damage."[22]

Flavonoids (Bioflavonoids, Vitamin P)

More than 5,000 flavonoids have been identified, with at least more than 60 in citrus fruits alone. Anthocyanins, a subgroup of flavonoids, accounts for the majority of yellow, red and blue pigmentation in foods. Another subgroup, formerly referred to as vitamin P, is called *bioflavonoids*, and includes citrin, rutin, hesperidin, quercitin, myricetin and kampferol, and others (the latter three are known to help prevent cataracts and protect foods from oxidation). Certain other bioflavonoids such as nobiletin and tangerin, can stimulate enzymes that detoxify our body from drugs and carcinogenic chemicals.[23]

Bioflavonoids are regarded as substances in foods concerned with the maintenance of a normal state of walls of small blood vessels. *Dorlands Medical Dictionary* explains, "Flavonoids are grouped in order of increasing oxidation state: catechins; leucoanthocyanidins and flavanones, flavanols, flavones, and anthocyanidins; and flavonols."[24] Acting as antioxidants, flavonoids guard against the oxygen-robbing effects of free radicals that are present in environmental pollutants as well as within the human body (generated as a result of biochemical functions). "Flavonoids can stabilize

[22] American Academy of Nutritional Sciences; Goldberg, et.al.

[23] Reuben, C.A., Carolyn and Joan Priestley, M.D., *Essential Supplements for Women*, Perigee Books, New York, 1988, page 88.

[24] *Dorlands Illustrated Medical Dictionary*, 26th Edition, W.B. Saunders, Philadelphia,1985, page 509.

connective tissue and capillaries, and seem to work together with vitamin C in this regard. They also decrease [actually aid the process of] inflammation by several mechanisms. They inhibit the infiltration of immune cells that cause inflammation (neutrophils). They block enzymes that generate inflammatory prostaglandins and leukotrienes, fatty acid derivatives with hormone-like qualities, and they desensitize mast cells, a type of immune cell embedded in tissues that release inflammatory agents like histamine when they encounter a foreign invader. Various flavonoids decrease the ability of platelets to form dangerous blood clots. Flavonoids can either activate or inhibit detoxification enzymes of the liver that help dispose of wastes and toxic materials."[25]

Phytoestrols

Robert Ronzio, Ph.D., author of *The Encyclopedia of Nutrition & Good Health*, defines phytoestrols as plant-based substances which mimic the influences of the female sex hormone estrogen. Thus, it is believed that phytoestrols (also called phytoestrogens) may inhibit some cancers, including breast cancer. Soybeans, lentils, various legumes and peas are sources of phytoestrogens. Phytoestrogens are believed to support estrogen functions in the body. Estrogens cause cells in certain parts of the body to proliferate—to increase in number. They promote the cellular health of the vagina, uterus, pelvis, breasts and fatty tissues deposited in areas such as the thighs and hips.

Plant estrogens, states nutritional researcher Mindy Kurzer, University of Minnesota, "'are thousands of times weaker than natural estrogen. But they also circulate in the blood at levels thousands of times higher than natural estrogen.'"[26] The net result is that, even in micro-amounts, they offer a beneficial effect.

---

[25] Ronzio, page 350.
[26] Schardt, David, "Phytoestrogens for Menopause," *Nutrition Action Health Letter*, January/February 2000, Volume 27, Number 1, Center for Science in the Public Interest, page 8-9.

It is speculated that lower incidents in menopause-related symptomatology in Asia may be directly related to diets with greater amounts of phytoestrogen plants.

One report explains,

> "After menopause, estrogen levels drop, and dietary sources of estrogen may have an important role in the female body. In Japan, where phytoestrogen rich soybeans are a common part of the diet (although only around 4-5 grams per day are eaten, on the average), only 10-15 percent of women experience menopause symptoms, where 80-85 percent of European and North American women (and who eat a standard western diet) *do* experience symptoms at menopause.

> Some people assert that the early onset of puberty in girls in the West is 'caused by' the soya component of food. However, Asian girls, who eat similar or higher amounts of soy do *not* have early puberty. The much simpler and more obvious explanation is that the calorie rich Western diet *both* brings the body mass up to the critical 45kg that allows the onset of menstruation much earlier, *and* that the intricate glucose metabolism/sex hormone synthesis mechanism has been made potentially partly dysfunctional by evolutionary inappropriate dietary composition and it's concomitant unusual metabolic pathways (unusual compared to the biochemical composition of the food that was presented to our metabolic pathways over the last million years or so).

> In a recent study menopausal women were asked to supplement their diet with a phytoestrogen containing food—soy flour, flax seed oil, or red clover sprouts. The soy flour and flax oil (only) significantly prevented the vaginal mucosa from thinning and drying; but the effect of eliminating these foods caused the mucosa to return to the previous menopausal thinning and drying.

In yet another study, post-menopausal women with bad blood fat profiles were split into two groups, with one group given bread and muffins made with flax seeds, the other group foods made with sunflower seeds. After six weeks, they switched seeds for another six weeks. The flaxseed lowered the 'bad' LDL cholesterol by 25 mg/dL (a 14.7% reduction) and levels of a protein called 'lipoprotein (a)', by 0.07 mm/L. Artificial estrogen supplements lower levels of this particular protein, 'lipoprotein (a)', but this is the first study to demonstrate that diet can also reduce the levels, possibly due to the weakly estrogenic lignans.[27]

As "weak estrogens," having 1/50,000 the potency of a dose of synthetic estrogen, certain bioflavonoids help to regulate estrogen levels, as they contain compounds that bind to estrogen receptors and act as a substitute form of estrogen in the body—especially beneficial when the body is no longer producing adequate supplies.

The controversy over soy as a "good" food is a raging debate. According to several researchers, including Gregory Burke and colleagues, Wake Forest University, North Carolina, researchers in Italy, and scientists at Tufts University, studies with soy have not yielded significant results proving the benefits of soy products to relieve menopausal symptoms. On the other hand is the double-blind study conducted in Italy alluding to the fact that soy protein reduces menopausal hot flashes. In this placebo-controlled study of 104 postmenopausal women seeking medical treatment for severe hot flashes, "Results showed that soy protein was significantly more effective than the placebo in reducing the frequency of hot flashes. Fifty-one women took 60g a day of isolated soy protein, and 53 women took a placebo. Forty patients in the soy group and 39 on the placebo completed

---

27 *"Hormone regulatory effect in women"*, Natural food-Grains Beans and Seeds, The Natural Food Hub, 2000 UHIS

the trial. By the third week, women taking soy had a 26 percent reduction in hot flashes, a percentage that increased to 33 percent by the fourth week. By the end of the study, those taking soy had a 45 percent reduction in hot flashes, compared to 30 percent of women taking the placebo."[28] This study showed that soy protein "markedly diminishes" moderate-to-severe hot flashes, but showed that other menopausal symptoms—anxiety, headaches, muscle aches and insomnia appears unaffected by soy supplementation. Evelyn Leigh, Herb Research Foundation, explains, "Soy foods contain phytoestrogens, compounds that have been shown to have both estrogenic and antiestrogenic properties and that may help protect against certain cancers, especially breast cancer. Phytoestrogens are much gentler and less powerful than synthetic estrogens. The authors of the Italian study note that although the 45 percent reduction in hot flashes they report is impressive, research has shown that treatment with synthetic estrogens can reduce hot flashes by as much as 83 percent." However, the concerns with synthetic estrogens used in hormone replacement therapy, Leigh noted, include the "risk of breast cancer and venous thromboembolism, a dangerous blood-clotting disorder."[29]

Soy Foods, Phytoestrogens & Phytates

Nutrition writer David Schardt claims, "The food that is richest by far in phytoestrogens is soybeans. A typical three-ounce serving of tofu, for example, contains about 23 milligrams of isoflavones (the major group of phytoestrogens). About a half-cup of shelled peanuts, on the other hand, has less than a tenth of a milligram. Menopausal supplements made from

---

[28] Leigh, Evelyn, Herb Reseaerch Foundation, "Soy protein reduces hot flashes,"*Herbs for Health*, September/October 1998, re: P. Albertazzi, et.al., "The effect of dietary soy supplementation on hot flashes," *Obstetrics & Gynecology*, 1998, 91 (1): 6-11.
[29] ibid.

herbs like black cohosh, red clover, and dong quai may contain soy-like levels of plant estrogens."[30]

Although soy foods are frequently touted as beneficial to the female hormonal system, providing phytoestrogens, to be fair we should look at the negative side of soy. Some researchers argue that, because most soy products (as well as cereal grains and other plant foods) are cooked, heated, milled or otherwise denatured in processing, much of the phyto-estrogen (and other nutrient) benefit may be lost. Worse yet, it is argued that in the processing of soy (non-fermented such as tofu and soymik, with isoflavones in an altered state), carcinogens and "anti-nutrients" are produced.[31] Further, the destruction of certain enzymes (e.g., phytase) may allow phytic acid inherent in many foods to survive digestion and inhibit mineral absorption.

Phytic Acids & Cereal Grains

Researchers studying the primitive, Paleolithic diet are questioning whether human beings are "equipped" to consume many of the cereal grains that are now in the diet, especially in consideration of food processing which adversely affect vital enzyme activity. Researcher Staffan Lindeberg writes,

"Whole meal cereals and other seeds have in their shells **phytic acid which strongly binds to minerals like calcium, iron, zinc and magnesium to form insoluble salts, phytates.** It is well known that whole meal cereals by this mechanism decrease the

---

[30] ibid.

[31] Fallon, MA, Sally and Mary Enig, Ph.D., *The Ploy of Soy: A Debate on Modern Soy Products*, Price Pottenger Nutrition Foundation, Health Freedom News, Sept 1995, p. 5, citing: Katz, Solomon H, "Food and Biocultrual Evolution: A Model for the Investigation of Modern Nutritional Problems," *Nutritional Anthropology*, Alan R. Liss, Inc., 1987, p. 50.

absorption of such minerals. There is apparently no [genetic/evolutionary] adaptation to a habitual high intake of phytic acid which is an important contributing cause of iron deficiency in third world countries and possibly in the western world. It is also an important cause of mineral deficiency in vegetarians. [Researchers] found back in the 30s that young dogs got rickets when they were fed oatmeal. [They were] made aware of the calcium-binding effect of phytate and showed that phytate was the dietary factor responsible for inhibition of calcium absorption by oatmeal as well as the induction of rickets in dogs. McCance and Widdowson found adverse effects of bread prepared from high-extraction wheat flour on retention of essential metals by humans. They also showed that destruction of phytate improved retention of calcium. Substantial evidence...later firmly established this negative impact of phytate. Not even rats seem to be fully adapted to graminivorous diets since phytate adversely affects mineral absorption in them as well.

In the archaeological record, rickets is rare or absent in preagricultural human skeletons, while the prevalence increases during medieval urbanization and then explodes during industrialism [19]. In the year 1900, an estimated 80-90 percent of Northern European children were affected. This can hardly be explained only in terms of decreasing exposure to sunlight and decreased length of breast-feeding. An additional possible cause is a secular trend of increasing intake of phytate since cereal intake increased during the Middle Ages...and since old methods of reducing the phytate content such as malting soaking, scalding, fermentation, germination and sourdough baking may have been lost during the agrarian revolution and industrialism by the emergence of large-scale cereal processing. The mentioned methods reduce the amount of phytic acid by use of phytases, enzymes which are also present in cereals. These enzymes are easily destroyed during industrial cereal processing.[32]

With soy and other plant foods, we see how a real, whole and natural food can be converted into a potentially harmful food by making such foods incomplete, or fractionated. Food researchers Sally Fallon, MA and Mary Enig, Ph.D. elucidate on how soy products may render one unhealthy:

> The production of soy milk is relatively simple. [T]he beans are first soaked in an alkaline solution. The pureed solution is then heated to about 115 degrees C in a pressure cooker. This method destroys most (but not all) of the anti-nutrients but has the unhappy side effect of so denaturing the proteins that they become very difficult to digest and much reduced in effectiveness.

---

[32] Lindeberg, Staffan, "Cereal Grains," Paleolithic Diet Symposium; Jun 1997, citing:1.Sandstead HH. Fiber, phytates, and mineral nutrition. Nutr Rev 1992; 50: 30-1. 2.Walker ARP, Walker BF I. I. Fiber, phytic acid, and mineral metabolism. Nutr Rev 1992; 50: 246-7. 3. Spivey Fox MR, Tao S-H. Antinutritive effects of phytate and other phosphorylated derivatives. In: Hathcock JN, ed. Nutritional Toxicology. New York: Academic Press, 1989: 59-96. vol 3). 4. Harland BF. Dietary fibre and mineral bioavailability. Nutr Res Rev 1989; 2: 133-47. 5. Rossander L, Sandberg A-S, Sandstr=F6m B. The influence of dietary fibre on mineral absorption and utilisation. In: Schweizer TF, Edwards CA, ed. Dietary fibre-a component of food. Nutritional function in health and disease. London: 1992: 6. Sandberg AS, Hasselblad C, Hasselblad K, Hulten L. The effect of wheat bran on the absorption of minerals in the small intestine. Br J Nutr 1982; 48: 185-91. 7.Morris ER. Phytate and dietary mineral bioavailability. In: Graf E, ed. Phytic acid: Chemistry and applications. Minneapolis: Pilatus Press, 1986: 57-76. vol 4). 8. Brune M, Rossander L, Hallberg L. Iron absorption: no intestinal adaptation to a high-phytate diet. Am J Clin Nutr 1989; 49: 542-5. 9. Hallberg L, Rossander L, Skanberg AB. Phytates and the inhibitory effect of bran on iron absorption in man. Am J Clin Nutr 1987; 45: 988-96. 10. Harland BF, Smith SA, Howard MP, Ellis R, Smith JJ. Nutritional status and phytate:zinc and phytate x calcium:zinc dietary molar ratios of lacto-ovo vegetarian Trappist monks: 10 years later. J Am Diet Assoc 1988; 88: 1562-6. 11.Ellis R, Kelsay JL, Reynolds RD, Morris ER, Moser PB, Frazier CW. Phytate:zinc and phytate X calcium:zinc millimolar ratios in self-selected diets of

Americans, Asian Indians, and Nepalese. J Am Diet Assoc 1987; 87: 1043-7. 12.Gibson RS. Content and ioavailability of trace elements in vegetarian diets. Am J Clin Nutr 1994; 59(5 Suppl): 1223S-1232S. 13. Mellanby E. A story of nutrition research.Baltimore: Williams & Wilkins Co, 1950 14.Bruce H, Callow R. Cereals and rickets. The role of inositolhexaphosphoric acid. Biochem J 1934; 28: 517-28. 15. Harrison D, Mellanby E. Phytic acid and the rickets-producing action of cereals. Biochem J 1934; 28: 517-28 16. McCance R, Widdowsos E. Mineral metabolism of healthy adults on white and brown bread dietaries. j Physiol 1942; 101: 44-85. 17. McCance R, Edgecombe C, Widdowson E. Mineral metabolism of dephy-tinized bread. J Physiol 1942; 101: 18. Fairweather TS, Wright AJ. The effects of sugar-beet fibre and wheat bran on iron and zinc absorption in rats. Br J Nutr 1990; 64: 547-52. 19. Stuart-Macadam PL. Nutritional deficiency diseases: a survey of scurvy, rickets, and iron-deficiency anemia. In: Is=E7an MY, Kennedy KAR, ed=.Reconstruction of life from the human skeleton. New York: Wiley-Liss, 1989: 201-22.; 20. Gibbs D. Rickets and the crippled child: an historical perspective [see comments]. J R Soc Med 1994; 87: 729-32. 21. Hernigou P. Historical overview of rickets, osteomalacia, and vitamin D. Rev Rhum Engl Ed 1995; 62: 261-70. 22. Sandberg AS. The effect of food processing on phytate hydrolysis and availability of iron and zinc. Adv Exp Med Biol 1991; 289: 499-508. 23. Svanberg U, Sandberg A-S. improved iron availability in weaning foods using germination and fermenta-tion. In: Southgate DAT, Johnson IT, =46enwick GR, ed. Nutrient Availability: Chemical and biological aspects. Cambridge: Cambridge University press, 1989: 179-81. 24. Larsson M, Sandberg A-S. Phytate reduction in bread containing oat flour, oat bran or rye bran. *J Cereal Sci* 1991; 14: 141-9. 25. Navert B, Sandstrom B, Cederblad A. Reduction of the phytate content of bran by leavening in bread and its effect on zinc absorption in man. *Br J Nutr* 1985; 53: 47-53. 26. Caprez A, Fairweather TS. The effect of heat treatment and particle size of bran on mineral absorption in rats. *Br J Nutr* 1982; 48: 467-75. 27. Sandberg A-S. Food processing influencing iron bioavailability. In: Hallberg L, Asp N-G, ed. Iron Nutrition in Health and Disease. London: John Libbey, 1996: 349-58. 28. Sandstrom B. Food processing and trace element supply. In: Somogyi JC, Muller HR, ed. Nutritional Impact of Food Processing. Bibl Nutr Dieta. Basel: Karger, 1989: 165-72. 29. Andersson H, Navert B, Bingham SA, Englyst HN, Cummings JH. The effects of breads containing similar amounts of phytate but different amounts of wheat bran on calcium, zinc and iron balance in man. Br J Nutr 1983; 50: 503-10.

The phytate content remains in soy milk to block the uptake of essential minerals [including zinc which is especially needed by growing babies and children, but used freely in baby formulas]. In addition, the alkaline soaking solution produces a carcinogen, lysinealine, and reduces the cystine content, which is already low in the soybean. Lacking cystine, the entire protein complex of the soybean becomes useless…Most soy products that imitate American food items, including baby formulas and some brands of soy milk, are made with **soy protein isolate**, that is the soy protein isolated from the carbohydrate and fatty acid components that naturally occur in the [soy]bean. Soybeans are first ground and subjected to high temperature and solvent extraction processes to remove the oils. The resultant defatted meal is then mixed with an alkaline solution and sugars in a separation process to remove the oils. The resultant defatted meal is then separated using an acid wash. Finally the resultant curds are neutralized in an alkaline solution and spray dried at high temperatures to produce high protein powder. This is a highly refined product in which both vitamin and protein quality are compromised…Soy protein isolate is the main ingredient of soy-based infant formulas. Along with trypsin inhibitors, these formulas have a high phytate content. Use of soy formula has caused zinc deficiency in infants [vital for growth, sexual function, liver health, brain development, intelligence levels, hormonal system and more].[33]

Thus, the American public consuming such processed soy products are receiving a far different food than the highly regarded fermented soy products of traditional cultures. The reader may contact the Price Pottenger

---

[33] Fallon, MA, Sally and Mary Enig, Ph.D., *The Ploy of Soy: A Debate on Modern Soy Products*, Price Pottenger Nutrition Foundation, Health Freedom News, September 1995

Nutrition Foundation for a more complete exposé on the pros and cons of soy products.

The moral of the story is: "Don't be so quick to blame any plant as being unhealthful without first determining whether it was altered and rendered harmful by means of processing."

Phytoestrogens & Alfalfa

Alfalfa (*medicago sativa*) is now receiving praise as an excellent, nutrient-dense food, recognized as a source of minerals, vitamins, chlorophyll and antioxidants.

One of the most promising new uses for *Medicago* appears to be in the treatment of endocrine imbalance. Its hormonal activity was first noted in veterinary medicine, where it was observed that animals grazing on alfalfa at times developed traits analogous to those animals treated with synthetic estrogens. Investigators were able to identify **several hormonally active compounds in** *Medicago*, **the most important group of these being the phytoestrogens.** These compounds are not true estrogens, yet they possess molecular structures similar enough to estrogen to bind to estradiol receptors. *Medicago* contains three major phytoestrogens: *coumestrol, genistein* and *formonetin*; and two less important ones, *diadzein* and *biochanin.*[34]

[34] Reilly, ND, Paul, Clinical Application: Medicago sativa extracts, Volume 1, Number 1, 1999, citing 1. Martin P. et al. Phytoestrogen interaction with estrogen receptor in human breast cancer cells. Endocrinology 1978:103; 1860; 2. Cheng E, et al. Estrogenic activity of some isoflavone derivatives. Science 1954;129:575; 3. FolmanY, et al. The interaction in the immature mouse of potent oesterogens with coumestrol, genestein and other utero-vaginotropic compounds of low potency. J Endocrinology 1966;34:215; 4. Shemish M, et al Affinity of rabbit uterine oestradiol receptor for phyto-oesterogens and its use in a competitive protein-binding radioassay for plasma coumesterol. J Reprod Pert 1972;29:1; 5. Noteboom W. et al. Estrogenic effect of genistein and coumestrol

Coumestrol is the most hormonally active of the group, with a relative estrogenic activity five percent that of estradiol. This is followed by genistein with one percent, and formonetin with.01 percent activity. The amount of estrogenic activity of a particular batch of *medicago* can vary greatly; the activity is highest in the full blooming and seeding stages, and lowest in the spring. The practical importance of the phytoestrogens lies with their ability to alter the biological response to endogenous estrogen. Estradiol receptors will bind to a diverse group of chemical compounds, including other steroids, isoflavones and phytoestrogens. **When phytoestrogens bind to estrogen receptors on cells, they translocate to the nucleus and stimulate cell growth in a manner similar to estradiol.** Despite the apparently weak relative binding capacity of the phytoestrogens, they can have significant hormonal effects. **This is due to their lower affinity for the serum estrogen binding proteins, thus resulting in a net effect of enhancing the concentration of available phytoestrogen at the target tissue sites.**

The relative weakness of their estrogenic action means that these compounds will have an "alterative" or "balancing" effect. Thus, **phytoestrogens may be used therapeutically in both**

diacetate. Endocrinology 1963;73:736; 6. Adler J. et al. Anti-oestrogenic activity in alfalfa. Vet Record 1962;74:1148; 7. Bickhoff E, et al. Estrogenic activity of coumestrol and related compounds. Arch Biochem Biophys 1960;88:262; 8. Emmons CW, et al. Oestrogenic, anti-oestrogenic and antifertility activities of various compounds. J Reprod Pert 1965;9:277; 9. Schutt D, et al. Steroid and phyto-oestrogen binding to sheep uterine receptors in vitro. J Endocrin 1972;52:299; 10. Livingston L. Forage plant estrogens. J Tox Envir Health 1978;4:301; 11. Morley J. et al. A prolactin inhibitory factor with immunocharacteristics similar to thytropin releasing factor (TRH) is present in rat pituitary tumors (Gh3 &W5), testicular tissue, and a plant material, alfalfa. Biochem Biophys Res Comm 1980;96:47; 12. Jackson I. Abundance of immunoreactive thytropin releasing hormone-like material in the alfalfa plant. Endocrinology 1981;108;344

hypoestrogenism and hyperestrogenism states. It is precisely this quality that makes them so useful therapeutically, especially in a naturopathic setting.

In conditions of hypoestrogenism, the plant estrogens will bind directly to estrogen receptors and provide a mild estrogenic effect. This is enhanced by the tendency of the phytoestrogens to concentrate in reproductive tissues, in preference to the serum proteins. This has been clearly demonstrated both in the field (feeding alfalfa to dairy cows can have effects similar to parenterally administered estrogens), and in the laboratory (uterine weight assays show effects equivalent to estradiol when sufficient phytoestrogen was used). **This implies a useful role for the phytoestrogens as adjuncts in the treatment of hypoestrogenic conditions, including hot flashes, menopausal vaginal atrophy and treatment or prevention of osteoporosis.**

These compounds are equally useful in conditions of hyper-estrogenism. The relatively weak-acting phytoestrogens will compete for binding sites, thus reducing the number of receptors available to the stronger endogenous estrogens and reducing net estrogenic stimulation. This is most useful in **estrogen excess conditions such as premenstrual syndrome, fibrocystic breasts, uterine leiyomyomas, and estrogen-responsive cancers of the breast and uterus.**

Phytoestrogens are not the only hormonally active compounds found in *Medicago* extracts. At least one author has identified an antiestrogenic compound distinct from the phytoestrogens. This compound is chloroform-soluable and reduces the estrogenic activity of phytoestrogens, diethylstilbestrol and estradiol. This compound appears to have a relative strength of approximately 12 percent that of the proestrogen activity of the phytoestrogens and would appear to have complementary effects desirable in the treatment of hyperestrogenism.[35]

Carotenoids

Carotenoids, discussed further under "Vitamin A," are antioxidant components of foods, including, but not limited to, alpha carotene and beta carotene. Carotenes are found in carrots, yams, cantaloupe, dandelion, wheat grass, squash and many other green and yellow vegetables; and are presumed to enhance the body's immune system by acting as antioxidants and feeding the liver the building blocks of vitamin A.

Indoles, Coumarins, Terpenes, et. al.

Indoles (not to be confused with the indoles that are produced by the decomposition of tryptophan in the intestines; or substances regarded as toxins) are found in cruciferous vegetables (cabbage family) such as cauliflower, rutabagas, turnips, broccoli, cabbage and Brussels sprouts. Indoles are a class of compounds with a structure resembling that of the amino acid tryptophan, and are believed to exhibit some anticancer action.

Coumarins are anti-coagulant food substances found in plants such as citrus fruits and tomatoes. Coumarins are believed to stimulate detoxification of the liver.

Organosulfur compounds include diallyl disulfide, S-allylcyssteine and others and are found in garlic, onions, leeks, shallots, chives and other so-called "sulfur foods." Much study has been made over garlic and its unique properties as an organosulfur food, including its abilities to destroy bacteria and inhibit high blood pressure. Garlic is widely used by natural healthcare practitioners in cases of high cholesterol, atherosclerosis, high blood pressure, athlete's foot, bronchiole infections, recurrent ear infections, parasites

---

[35] ibid

and vaginitis. Its active constituent is allicin and it contains other sulfur compounds including ajoene, allyl sulfides and vinyldithiins.

"Three reviews of double-blind studies in humans have found that garlic can lower blood cholesterol levels in adults by approximately ten percent. Garlic has been shown to be as effective as the drug bezafibrate in lowering cholesterol levels...Several double-blind studies also suggest it can prevent atherosclerosis."[36] In addition, "Human population studies show that eating garlic regularly reduces the risk of esophageal, stomach and colon cancer...Animal and test tube studies also show that garlic and its sulfur compounds inhibit the growth of different types of cancer—especially breast and skin tumors."[37]

It is speculated that organosufur compounds play a role in cancer suppression, by blocking carcinogens and suppressing carcinogenic changes in cells.

Terpenes are another form of phytochemical, and are found in citrus fruit, caraway seeds, licorice root and other fruits and vegetables. Terpenes are chiefly from essential oils, resins and other vegetable aromatic products. With subgroups of monoterpenes and triterpenes, terpenes also may block the action of carcinogens and inhibit hormone-related cancers.[38] Terpenes are long-chain lipids of great biochemical importance and include the photosynthetic pigment chlorophyll as well as the pigment retinal which absorbs light in the eyes.[39]

[36] Lininger, Jr., DC, Schuyler, and Alan R. Gaby, MD, et.al., *The Natural Pharmacy*, Healthnotes, Inc., 1999, page 426

[37] ibid.

[38] Ronzio, page 350.

[39] Raven, Peter H., Director, Missouri Botanical Garden; Engelmann Professor of Botany, Washington University, St. Louis, Missouri and George B Johnson, Professor of Biology, Washington University, St. Louis, Missouri : *Biology*, Third Edition Mosby-Year Book, Inc., Missouri, 1992, pages 49-50.

Yet another form of phytochemical is saponin, contained in soybeans, several vegetables and herbs. Saponins have been studied for their anti-cancer activity and in lowering high blood pressure and high cholesterol.

Lignans, found in flaxseed, wheat and barley are also cancer-defeating compounds of the phytochemical variety.

Isothiocyanates

A salt of isothiocyanic acid, an isothiocyanate food substance, is found in the cabbage family and possesses sulfur compounds said to "protect against some forms of cancer. Sulforaphane is one example. Isothiocyanates seem to act on detoxification mechanisms, thus speeding up the inactivation and disposal of potentially harmful compounds like pollutants from the body."[40]

Plant Pigments

Plant pigments are often spoken of as part of the whole food complex, yet these colorful components are rarely defined in terms of their value. To many species of animals and insects, the colors of plants make them attractive and recognizable for consumption. Plant color also provides camouflage from natural predators, and we know that certain colors attract and absorb the sun's rays to different degrees. Pigments also absorb energy and thereby offer this energy to the consumer, making pigmented plants (e.g., chlorophyll, carotenes) salubrious foods.

The orange pigment, beta carotene—best known of the plant color compounds—first caught researchers' eyes when population studies linked low rates of certain cancers with a high intake of fruits and vegetables containing lots of beta carotene. A current theory holds that cancer, heart disease, stroke, and other diseases

---

[40] Ronzio, page 351.

of aging result from cumulative damage to cells by free radicals—most of which our cells generate through ordinary metabolism. So nutrition and medical researchers are dissecting the fruits and vegetables consumed by healthy populations, looking for the best combinations to prevent such damage. What they are finding is that **fruits and vegetables contain hundreds of other pigments besides beta carotene**—as well as nonpigment compounds—that may play a role in preventing oxidative damage. [These other pigments are absent in isolated vitamin A and beta carotene supplements].

Studies to date suggest many pigmented plant chemicals, [phytochemicals], appear to maintain health by boosting the immune system, reducing inflammation and allergies, detoxifying contaminants and pollutants, and/or activating enzymes that block unbridled cell division. Fred Khachik, a chemist with ARS [Agricultural Research Service], points out that the diets of most people supply more of two other carotenoids—lutein and lycopene—than they do beta carotene.[41]

Chlorophyll

Many of our "green foods" are the source of important vitamin A precursors, as well as minerals and trace elements. Such substances, when fractionated or isolated from the green food, leave behind the very valuable chlorophyll component. Research is only just beginning to illuminate the value of chlorophyll as a healing agent, both topically and internally.

Dorland's Medical Dictionary defines chlorophyll as the green coloring matter of plants by which photosynthesis is accomplished. There are many types, including, but not limited to, bluish green found in oxygen-releasing

[41] McBride, Judy, *Agricultural Research/*, November 1996, ARS; Jean Mayer USDA Human Nutrition Research Center on Aging, Tufts University, Boston, MA

plants; a yellowish-green chlorophyll; chlorophyll found in marine algae; a red variety occurring in red algae; and bacteriochlorophylls found in phototropic bacteria. Water-soluble chlorophyll derivatives, "consisting mainly of the copper complex of the sodium and/or potassium salts of chlorophyll, are applied topically to the skin for deodorization, for enhancement of normal tissue repair, and for relief of itching in various skin lesions. Preparations of the derivatives for oral administration are used to deodorize certain necrotic, ulcerative lesions, to control fecal and urinary odors in colostomy, ileostomy or incontinence, and to deodorize urinary and fecal fistulas and breath and body odors not related to faulty hygiene."[42]

Chlorophyll is a lipid—a macromolecule of the oily or waxy class that is insoluble in water but soluble in oil, forming biologically important pigments. Plants and other photosynthetic organisms use chlorophyll to absorb light with great efficiency. In a complex system, the **captured light is converted into energy**.

Good dietary sources of chlorophyll include plant foods offering dark green leaves such as spinach, kale, lettuce and parsley. Within the last 20 years or so, chlorella, wheat grass, barley grass and algae (including spirulina) have gained added attention for their chlorophyll composition. Although many promises and anecdotal accounts tell of chlorophyll's miraculous role in healing, scant scientific literature exists on chlorophyll's curative abilities. However, some preliminary evidence may suggest that chlorophyll might be helpful in detoxifying cancer-promoting substances.[43]

In natural healthcare, chlorophyll is recommended in nutritional schedules in perles or whole, green food concentrated supplements for hormonal

---

[42] Dorland's. p. 211.

[43] Lininger, page 281; re: Gruskin B. Chlorophyll—its therapeutic place in acute and suppurative disea. *American Journal of Surgery* 1940; 49-56; ayatsu H, Negishi T, Arimoto S, et. al. Porphyrins as potential inhibitors against exposure to carcinogens and mutagens. *Mutat Res* 1993: 290; 79-85.

support, detoxification, blood platelet health and in the healing of wounds both internal and external. Author Ronald Seibold, MS writes,

"The action of chlorophyll on wounds has a unique feature. Most medicines become less effective with repeated use. In contrast, an initial application of chlorophyll makes a wound more sensitive to its healing benefits with repeated use...{Researcher} Dr. G.H. Collings considered chlorophyll to 'have the most constant and marked effect of all agents for stimulating cell proliferation and tissue repair.' Collings demonstrated that the healing time of wounds is shorter with chlorophyll therapy than with penicillin, vitamin D, sulfanilamide or no treatment.

Chlorophyll also accelerates wound healing by reducing hemagglutination and inflammation. When a tissue is injured, foreign substances in the blood generally cause blood cells to clump together. This limits the amount of nutrients available for repair of the injured tissue. When chlorophyll is administered to a wound, this clumping is reduced, so the lag time associated with tissue repair is shortened. Chlorophyll decreases swelling by reducing the synthesis of fibrin (the protein associated with blood clot formation). This gives chlorophyll a mild blood thinning, or heparin-like property, which can enhance the effectiveness of local immune defenses.

Chlorophyll has also been shown to be extremely effective in speeding the healing of peptic ulcers, wounds which develop internally in the gastrointestinal tract. Several studies document the use of chlorophyll in the treatment of ulcers resistant to more conventional therapies...In the Offenkrantz study, 20 of the 27 patients with chronic ulcers were relieved of pain and other symptoms in 24 to 27 hours. Complete healing of the damaged tissues, as demonstrated by x-ray examination, occurred in 20 of 24 cases within two to seven weeks. These reports include case descriptions of dramatic recoveries from severe, long standing problems...

European investigators report preliminary favorable results in the use of chlorophyll in the treatment of pancreatitis. The chlorophyll is thought to influence several enzymatic reactions which complicate this disease."[44]

---

[44] Seibold, page 45-47, citing: Smith, L 1955. The present status of topical chlorophyll therapy. *The NY State Journal of Medicine*, March, 1940; Chernomorsky, S and Segelman, A, 1988; Biological activities of chlorophyll derivatives, *New Jersey Medicine*, 85:669-673; Young, R and Beregi, J, 1980, Use of chlorophyllin in the care of geriatric patients, *Journal of the American geriatrics Society*, 28:46-47, 1980; Miller, J, Jackson, D and Collier, C, 1960. The inhibition of Russell's viper venom by the water-soluble derivatives of sodium-copper chlorophyllin. *American Journal of Surgery*, 99:48-49; Miller, J, Jackson, D and Collier, C, 1958, The inhibition of clotting by chlorophyllin, *American Journal of Surgery*, 95: 967-969; Sack, P and Barnard, R, 1955, Studies on the hemagglutinating and inflammation properties of exudate from nonhealing wounds and their inhibition by chlorophyll derivatives. *New York State Journal of Medicine*, October 15, 1955, p. 2952-2956.

THE POLITICS OF SUPPLEMENTS, VITAMINS & DRUGS

Politics enters into every field of endeavor in the modern world. We are reminded of the allegory of a political committee that once gathered to design a horse and, by the time they were through with the project, they produced a camel. Too often important decisions are made based not on the common good but rather economics motivated by corporate and personal agendas. As such, scientific studies and "findings" are often predicated not on the purposes of curing disease and eliminating suffering, but rather on profiteering. Here in America the pursuit of making money is an obses- sion—a national pastime yielding both good and bad. Many a noble out- come has resulted from inventors and scientists looking to make a better mousetrap. No doubt we have been uplifted by refrigerators, automobiles, surgical tools, construction materials, recreational equipment, emergency medical procedures and communications devices. Such creations have bene- fited manufacturers as well as the general public. However, it is also true that many innovations are not all they pretend to be. Through high-powered marketing campaigns and mass exploitation, the general public is made to accept, believe, utilize and crave many things that are not really good for them, but which make certain manufacturers financially successful. In the health arena, examples include refined wheat, refined sugars, artificial ingre- dients, preservatives, pesticides, and perhaps even vitamins, multivitamins and most drugs. None of these things are natural; even if they are *from* nature, they are no longer contained within the whole, natural entity. When we are told that they are life-enriching and life-sustaining, then the scales of balance are tipped away from the general public and in favor of the manufacturers—whom author Victor Herbert, M.D. has taken much criticism for calling "the vitamin pushers."

In lieu of receiving the healthiest forms of a food, vitamin or any other product, we as consumers are more apt to receive from manufacturers items and substances which are easiest, most convenient, fastest, best preserved and least expensive to produce and sell. The economics and politics of the day interfere with what is best for not only the seller, but also the buyer (patient, consumer). In this way, economics and politics may take precedence over environmental and health issues. Clearly, there is BIG money in the vitamin business (as mentioned, vitamin and mineral supplement sales are $6.4 billion per year); and the goal of vitamin manufacturers is to sell lots of vitamins, not to educate the public on the difference between a synthetic vitamin and a natural vitamin contained within the food complex. The overall idea seems to be to convince us that pills are superior to whole, natural, pure and raw foods—the nourishment that has sustained all life forms since the beginning of life on this planet. As long as people feel some sort of effect from a vitamin, and are convinced that they need this substance to the point where they will pay for a monthly supply, then manufacturers have achieved their goals. The health of the public is a secondary consideration, if it is a consideration at all. We too often forget that the cornerstone of modern economics, *caveat emptor* (buyer beware), should be applied to drugs, medical treatment, alternative healthcare and vitamins as well as any other marketed product or service.

Studies performed on the efficacy of vitamins, minerals and other nutrients are made on isolated (also called "fractionated") and synthetic components rather than on whole foods. Why? Economics. The purpose of conducting scientific studies in our modern world of science-meets-big business is primarily to ascertain the marketability and profitability of a given substance. Independent and private institutions conduct the most publicized scientific studies pertaining to vitamins, minerals and other food components. For a study to prove that vitamin C ascorbic acid, for example, helps alleviate flu symptoms is to prove that we should purchase vitamin C pills, which we do to the tune of billions of dollars each year.

In light of the prevailing economic picture, it is not difficult to imagine why studies on the nutrient properties contained within (and not fractionated away from) foods rarely make the headlines. Once we discover the wonders of a vitamin **still contained within** the food complex, who can make money on it other than food growers? Synthetic and fractionated vitamins and minerals are much easier to manufacture, preserve and sell. Thus, once foods and herbs are standardized (in terms of milligrams, micrograms, etc. by adding in isolated vitamins and minerals to the food or herb), scientists can predict their effect like any other drug-like substance, and promise results. On the other hand, with real, whole food, such predictability is implausible and dependent upon innumerous factors ranging from symptomatology to bioindividuality (to be discussed further). In nature, no two carrots, or oranges or potatoes will ever yield identical quantities of a specific vitamin or mineral. This fact of nature is used to argue against the efficacy of whole foods in fighting disease, feeding cells and providing immunity. But the naturalist will understand that the value of foods are not limited solely to vitamin and mineral content alone.

In this modern era, then, the practice of "nutrition" is a rare occurrence. Instead of practicing nutrition (the study and application of foods and their effect on illness and ability to promote health, energy and vitality), most "natural healthcare" practitioners actually practice pharmacology, using not foods, but rather isolated chemicals. As a result, there is probably more to learn from a farmer using medieval tools nestled in the Hunza valley than you can learn from a modern-day practitioner of nutrition or medicine. Instead of studying foods and their properties as part of the whole complex, the modern tendency is to study vitamins, minerals, amino acids and enzymes in the same way that a pharmacist studies various chemicals and compounds.

Naturalists argue that the most important question to consider for ourselves is not whether a vitamin or drug seems to work, but rather whether it works naturally, in accord with the principles of nature, in harmony with the body's biochemical and physiological functions, without upsetting natural systems, in micronutrient amounts (as opposed to unnaturally high potencies) and as a substance conceived by nature to rebuild a natural system (that of our own cellular structures).

ISOLATED VITAMINS COMPARED TO FOOD COMPLEX COFACTORS

Vitamins are substances found inside the original, natural food complex. A vitamin may be defined as "an organic compound needed in the diet in small amounts to promote and regulate the chemical reactions and processes of the body. An organic compound is classified as a vitamin if a lack of that compound in the diet results in symptoms that are relieved by addition of the substance to the diet. Although vitamins do not provide energy, many aid in the reactions that produce energy from carbohydrate, fat and protein."[45]

The word "vitamin" was coined by Polish biochemist Cashmir Funk who was best known for his work in curing the thiamine deficiency disease termed "beriberi." Using an extract of rice bran husks to achieve his successful nutritional treatment, Funk coined the term *vitamine*, thinking that the curative constituent in the food was an *amine* (a compound containing an amino group) that was vital to life (*vital+amine*).[46] Vitamins were designated with an alphabetical label as they were discovered for their properties. Some vitamins, including the B vitamins, were sub-designated with numerals (e.g., vitamin B_{12}) because, although originally assumed to be

---

[45] Smolin & Grosvenor, *Nutrition, Science & Applications*, Saunders College Publishing, 1994.
[46] ibid, page 248

one vitamin, individual B vitamins were eventually discovered to have different functions and structures. When vitamins were discovered not to be essential, they were dropped from the vitamin designation, leaving gaps in the alphabetical list. Some vitamins retain the name vitamin, yet are often considered something else altogether (such as vitamin F, the essential fatty acid, and vitamin P, now called flavonoids). Essentially, vitamins are categorized as being either water-or fat-soluble. Water-soluble vitamins include all but A, D, E and K. There are also substances which are termed *vitaminoids* and produce a vitamin-like activity; e.g., a bioflavonoid.

In many respects, vitamins are similar to hormones (vitamin D, for instance is considered a hormone). Both vitamins and hormones are carried by the bloodstream throughout the body to sites of particular need; and both are required by the body in "extremely small amounts."[47] Like hormones, vitamins do not create their own energy, although vitamins may combine with enzymes to control energy changes within the body. Unlike hormones, vitamins must be supplied in the diet; hormones are synthesized in the body itself.

VITAMINS ARE FOUND IN FOODS
ALONG WITH THEIR SYNERGISTS

Botanist and phytochemical researcher James Duke, Ph.D., retired, USDA (United States Department of Agriculture), states, "Vitamins and phytochemicals are better taken in their evolutionary context—as they occur in plants—not isolated and out of context." Duke established the landmark, monumentous Phytochemical Database for USDA that lists all the known chemical compounds in more than 1,000 edible plants, including the most common herbs and spices consumed. A worldwide authority on medicinal plants, Duke says there is mounting evidence that

---

[47] Sackheim, George and Ronald M. Schultz, *Chemistry for the Health Sciences*, The Macmillan Company, New York, 1973.

plant compounds work best in combination, not isolation, and believes this synergistic effect is an argument against "popping supplements."[48]

Echoing the same sentiment as Duke and others is Canadian medicinal plant researcher Keith Sterling, M.A., M.N.I.M.H., who writes: "Some plants contain over 170 different chemicals. These chemicals work together, and that is really the essence of the difference between allopathy and herbal medicine in its holistic approach. When pharmaceutical interests began to synthesize plant drugs, they eliminated the complete package that nature had presented us with. Among those 170 different constituents, you have buffers, tannins and mucilages. These things slow down or cushion the effect of the essential or active ingredients of the plants. But when we throw away nature's package, we are left with something that is very brutal and harsh on our systems."[49]

Vitamins do not exist in isolation in nature. That is, vitamins exist within foods. A food can contain a vitamin, but a vitamin does not contain the other cofactors found in foods, including a wide array of other nutrients and synergists naturally occurring along with vitamins in foods. Such co-factors include minerals, enzymes, coenzymes, amino acids, trace minerals, and energies and substances that may not have yet been identified by scientific method. As such, a vitamin by itself, either having been extracted from a real food, or a synthetically produced vitamin, is but a mere isolated substance that is no longer—or has never been—associated with a living, biochemical entity.

Ron Seibold, MS, author of *Cereal Grass: What's In It For You!* writes, "Foods contain hundreds of compounds which interact with each other in the foods themselves and in our digestive tracts and blood streams. The combinations of nutrients and their factors found in foods bear little

[48] Reavley, Nicola, *Vitamins, Etc.* and *Vitamin Update*, Bookman Press, Melbourne, Australia, 1999.

[49] Sterling, M.A., M.N.I.M.H., Keith, Medicinal Plants, Volume 15, Issue 1, January 1992.

resemblance to those found in the supplement pills in the health food stores, and are many times more complex. Low-dose supplements may fill some nutrient gaps, and mega-dose supplements may have therapeutic value, but neither can come close to replacing our need for food nutrition."[50] Seibold writes, "For fifty years, the beneficial effects of adding cereal grasses to the rations of test animals could not be duplicated by adding any or all of the known isolated chemical components of those foods. The results of many studies which demonstrate the value of green vegetables in the prevention of human disease cannot be explained in terms of the individual nutrients they are known to contain."[51]

In his article "Synergy," James Duke, Ph.D. wrote:

> For years I worked with the National Cancer Institute (NCI) and the United States Dept. Of Agriculture (USDA) collaborative cancer screening and collaborated with the National Institutes of Health (NIH) AIDS and Designer Food programs. I watched their scientists and contractors futilely follow their directed fractionations in search of the single super silver bullet compound in the herbal potpourri. It became clear that there were almost always, not one, but many closely related chemicals in a species, each of which contributed in slightly different ways to the activity of the whole herb. More often than not, these chemicals and their activities were synergistic, the whole herb being more active proportionately, than even the strongest single isolated ingredient. I cite the mayapple as an example. There's a billion-dollar anticancer drug made from one lignan that occurs in the mayapple root. But there are at least four different lignans in the root and they have been proven synergistic against the herpes virus. And just as I can now name you a hundred herbal

---

[50] Seibold, page 50.
[51] ibid, page 50.

alternatives that look very promising to beat their pharmaceutical competitors, I can cite a hundred cases, where I can re-read a scientific paper, and show that the whole plant extract (or a combination of the chemicals they studied) was proportionately more efficacious than any one of the chemicals alone, proving that either there was a synergy between the chemicals or that there was an as yet unstudied compound in the plant which had more activity than the compounds they studied. In either event it adds up to the **whole plant being better than the sum of its known parts.**....Remember modern agriculture, gradually modifying the chemical ratios in the plants we eat, has only been with us for some 10 millennia. And agriculture and even more so food processing take us farther and farther away from our evolutionary or "genetic" phytochemical ratios. Silver bullets, single solitary chemicals, are still even more likely to upset our genetic phytochemical ratios, and that's why they are more liable to have serious side effects than natural remedies our genes have experienced over the millennia.[52]

For the purposes of this study of vitamins, we have identified them by their individual names. However, the reader is urged to keep in mind that it is because of their synergists (in their natural states, quantities and ratios) vitamins are successful as nutrients in achieving health through their biochemical support.

[52] Duke, Ph.D. James, "Synergy," *Nature's Herbs Newsletter*, 1999.

VITAMIN A COMPLEX &
SYNERGISTIC COMPOSITION

Most vitamin A in capsule form, sold to the public as "vitamin A" is in the form of the synthetic vitamin A palmitate. In the whole food form, however, vitamin A is an extremely complex substance. Those who take vitamin A (or even beta carotene) as a synthetic or isolated vitamin supplement are failing to ingest the rest of the entire complex needed to perform infinite biochemical tasks.

"For thousands of years, liver has been used as a cure for night blindness but it was only in the early part of the 20th century that researchers discovered that it is a rich source of vitamin A, which is essential for healthy eyes. The first vitamin to be discovered, vitamin A was identified in 1913 when two American scientists showed that butter and egg yolk contained a substance which was necessary for healthy growth in rats. They called this substance 'fat soluble A.' (As with so many other food nutrients, despite the fact that vitamin A was the first vitamin to be discovered, its actions in the cells of our bodies are not well understood at a chemical level. However misunderstood how vitamins work at a biochemical level, it is the deficiency in specific vitamin-containing foods which makes their necessity and importance apparent.) By 1930 the structure of vitamin A was determined, and five years later it was found to be necessary for normal vision."[53]

---

[53] American Society of Nutritional Science: Britton, G. (1995) *Structure and properties of carotenoids in relation to function*. FASEB J. 9: 1551-1558 ; and Krinsky, N.I. (1993) *Actions of carotenoids in biological systems*. Ann. Rev. Nutr. 13: 561-587.

How 'Complex' is Vitamin A?

"Vitamin A consists of three biologically active molecules: retinol, retinal (retinaldehyde) and retinoic acid. Each of these compounds are
derived from the plant precursor molecule, b-carotene (a member of a
family of molecules known as *carotenoids*). Beta-carotene, which consists
of two molecules of retinal linked at their aldehyde ends, is also referred
to as the *provitamin* form of vitamin A [because the body can manufacture vitamin A from carotenoids). Ingested b-carotene is cleaved in the
lumen of the intestine by *b-carotene dioxygenase* to yield retinal. Retinal is
reduced to retinol by *retinaldehyde reductase*, an NADPH requiring
enzyme within the intestines. Retinol is esterified [combined with an
alcohol with elimination of a molecule of water] to palmitic acid and
delivered to the blood via *chylomicrons* [basically, fatty substances used by
the body to transport long-chain fats and cholesterol from the intestine].
The uptake of chylomicron remnants by the liver results in delivery of
retinol to this organ for storage as a lipid ester within lipocytes [fat cells].
Transport of retinol from the liver to extrahepatic [outside the liver] tissues occurs by binding of hydrolyzed retinol to a retinol binding protein
(RBP). The retinol-RBP complex is then transported to the cell surface
within the Golgi and secreted. Within extrahepatic tissues retinol is
bound to cellular retinol binding protein (CRBP). Plasma transport of
retinoic acid is accomplished by binding to albumin."[54]

Gene Control Exerted by Retinol and Retinoic Acid

Within cells, retinol and retinoic acid bind to specific receptor proteins.
Following binding, the receptor-vitamin complex interacts with specific
sequences in several genes involved in growth and differentiation and
affects expression of these genes. In this capacity, retinol and retinoic acid

---

[54] King, Ph.D., Michael W., Department of Medical Biochemistry, Terre
Haute Center for Medical Education, Indiana State University, November 1999.

are considered hormones of the steroid/thyroid hormone superfamily of proteins. (Vitamin D also acts in a similar capacity.) Several genes whose patterns of expression are altered by retinoic acid are involved in the earliest processes of embryogenesis (the process of embryo development) including the differentiation of germ (substances that eventually form into organs, etc.) layers, the formation of organs, and limb development. [55]

Retinol also functions in the synthesis (formation) of certain glycoproteins and mucopolysaccharides necessary for mucous production and normal growth regulation. This is accomplished by converting retinol to retinyl phosphate.

Food Sources of Vitamin A

"While the vitamin A we obtain from food comes in many different forms, these can be divided into two main types—pre-formed vitamin A and provitamin A. Pre-formed vitamin A which is often in the form of retinol or retinal, is found in foods of animal origin such as liver and butter. Provitamin A is the name given to around 50 compounds in a group of plant pigments known as carotenes (or carotenoids), with beta carotene being the best known of these. This is because these compounds can be turned into vitamin A in the body. Both pre-formed vitamin A and provitamin A are fat soluble."

"There are over 600 carotenoids in nature. Carotenoids generally contain a conjugated polyene structure which is efficient at absorbing light, and are the major yellow and red pigments in many fruits and vegetables. Beta-carotene...and alpha-carotene are responsible for the orange color of carrots, and lycopene for the red color of tomatoes; astaxanthin imparts a red or pink color to lobsters and salmon. The term "carotene" refers to carotenoids which contain only carbon and hydrogen (e.g. beta-carotene, alpha-carotene, lycopene), while the term "xanthophylls" refers

---

[55] ibid.

to compounds which contain hydroxyl groups (lutein, zeaxanthin, beta-cryptoxanthin) or keto groups (canthaxanthin) or both (astaxanthin)."[56]

Vitamin A is found in fish liver oils, butter, milk and (to a lesser extent) in kidneys, fat and muscle meats. Vitamin A occurs naturally only in foods of animal origin, but the body converts certain carotenoids, especially beta carotene, to vitamin A. Only 50 of the more than 500 naturally occurring carotenoids have provitamin A activity. Provitamin A is a precursor (building block) of vitamin A and is found in yellow fruits and vegetables including peaches, carrots, apricots, squash, and sweet potatoes. Provitamin A can be converted into vitamin A within the body. As with any vitamin found in its original food complex, vitamin A is made up of several different components and is made to work as a nutrient not only by being intact with its other components, but also as it exists alongside other nutrients (minerals, trace mineral activators, etc.). Vitamin A is a family of compounds that includes retinol, retinal and the carotenoids. Therefore, it is important to consider that vitamin A is not an isolated substance, but rather "the name given to **a group of compounds** which have certain actions in the body."[57]

Chemists define vitamin A as an alcohol of high molecular weight. Two different forms include vitamin A_1 and vitamin A_2, with vitamin A_2 containing one additional double bond in the (molecular) ring.[58] The potency of vitamin A_2 is said to be only 40 percent of that of vitamin A_1. As a precursor (provitamin A), one molecule of beta carotene produces two molecules of vitamin A_1. Alpha and gamma carotene yield only one molecule of vitamin A_1 because those compounds are not symmetrical as is beta-carotene.[59]

[56] American Society for Nutritional Sciences: Britton, G. (1995) *Structure and properties of carotenoids in relation to function. FASEB J.* 9: 1551-1558 ; and Krinsky, N.I. (1993) *Actions of carotenoids in biological systems. Ann. Rev. Nutr.* 13: 561-587.
[57] ibid.
[58] Sackheim, page 427.
[59] ibid, page 429.

Vitamin A is necessary for the growth and repair of many body cells including those of bones, teeth, collagen and cartilage. It is also essential for *cell differentiation*, a "process whereby cells change to take on different structures and functions; for instance, when one cell becomes a liver cell, whereas another becomes a red blood cell. Vitamin A's role in cell differentiation is probably related to its ability to interact with a cell's DNA to turn on and off various cellular functions. The role of vitamin A in cell differentiation is important in the maintenance of epithelial (the covering of internal and external surfaces of the body, including the lining of vessels and other small cavities) tissue, reproduction and immunity."[60]

Thus vitamin A plays a central role in tissue development and maintenance. Deficiency of vitamin A may cause epithelial tissues of the membranes in the eyes, digestive tract (esp. intestinal mucosa), respiratory tract and genitourinary tract (esp. germinal epithelium of ovaries and testes) to harden and shrink. This hardening, known as *keratinization*, has been attributed to many types of diseases, including colds, pneumonia and so-called respiratory infections—all related to the drying out of membranes. Keratinization leads to scaliness of the skin, failure of growth in young animals, failure of reproduction and corneal opacity. Keratinization may cause eye dryness, with malfunction of tear ducts. Medical findings attribute *xerophthalmia* to vitamin A deficiency, a condition in which the cornea becomes cloudy and fails to allow light to pass through.

Retinoic acid maintains differentiation of epithelial cells such as skin, lung, and intestinal tissue, but this form of vitamin A cannot be used in vision.[61]

Night blindness is an early symptom of vitamin A deficiency. The cause is said to be due to a subsequent lack of visual purple (rhodopsin) in the

[60] Smolin, page 259.
[61] Olson, J.A. (1994) *Vitamin A, retinoids, and carotenoids. In: Modern Nutrition in Health and Disease* (Shils, M.E., Olson, J.A. & Shike, M., eds), 8th ed., pp. 287-307, Lea & Febiger, Philadelphia, PA Sporn, M.B., Roberts, A.B. & Goodman, D.S. (eds.) (1994) *The Retinoids*, 2nd ed. Raven Press, New York, NY.

retina which depends on vitamin A for regeneration. Vitamin A is used by the eyes to synthesize the light-sensitive retinal pigments used by the rods and cones for vision. The rods and cones of the eye are nerve receptors excited by light. These cells change the light energy into neuronal signals that are transmitted into the brain.[62]

"It has been estimated that 0.5 million children in the world become blind each year; 70 percent of these are due to vitamin A deficiency. Over half of these blind children die from malnutrition and associated illnesses."[63]

Delving deeper into the specific role of the vitamin A complex in relation to vision, Michael King, Ph.D., Indiana State University Department of Medical Biochemistry, writes: "Photoreception in the eye is the function of two specialized cell types located in the retina; the rod and cone cells. Both rod and cone cells contain a photoreceptor pigment in their membranes. The photosensitive compound of most mammalian eyes is a protein called opsin to which is covalently coupled an aldehyde of vitamin A. The opsin of rod cells is called *scotopsin*. The photoreceptor of rod cells is specifically called *rhodopsin* or visual purple. This compound is a complex between scotopsin and the 11-cis-retinal (also called 11-cis-retinene) form of vitamin A."[64]

Other Uses for Vitamin A

A deficiency of vitamin A has been linked to at least one type of sterility, caused when epithelial cells of the genital system fail to make use of this required vitamin for reproductive function. In its role in cell development and cell differentiation, adequate vitamin A helps ensure that changes occurring in cells and tissues during fetal development take place normally. It is theorized to be involved in cell-to-cell communication.[65]

---

[62] Guyton, M.D., Arthur C., *Function of the Human Body*, W. B. Saunders Company, Philadelphia, 1974

[63] Olson.

[64] King.

[65] Reavley, 1998.

Vitamin A deficiency has also been linked to deformities of the teeth. Early symptoms include follicular hyperkeratinosis, increased susceptibility to infection and cancer, and anemia equivalent to iron-deficient anemia.[66]

Scientists claim that vitamin A is 'the anti-infective vitamin,' enabling body surfaces to act as barriers to invading micro-organisms and toxins. Biochemically, vitamin A stimulates and enhances many immune functions including antibody response and the activity of various white blood cells such as T helper cells and phagocytes. This immune-enhancing function is said to promote healing of infected tissues and an increased resistance to infection.

Vitamin A has antioxidant activity and plays a role in protecting against free radical damage contributing to many common diseases. Additionally, vitamin A is involved in iron metabolism and storage.

Because vitamin A is stored in the liver, and is fat soluble, the presence of fat and bile in the intestines is necessary for vitamin A absorption. Vitamin A is joined to fatty acids in the intestinal lining, combined with other substances, and transported to the liver, where 90 percent of the body's vitamin A is stored. Around 80 to 90 percent of vitamin A in the diet is absorbed, although this is reduced in older people and those who have trouble absorbing fat, such as pancreatitis, celiac disease and cystic fibrosis sufferers, who may run the risk of vitamin A deficiency.[67] Therefore, bile deficiency, often associated with liver and gall bladder problems, may lead to vitamin A deficiency. In this regard, the supplementation with fractionated or synthetic forms of vitamin A, without sufficient bile activity, may contribute to toxicity.

Vitamin A has long been a subject of study in regard to cancer treatment and prevention, especially in lung cancer where the vitality of the cells lining the respiratory system is integral to health, immunity and function. In

[66] King.
[67] ibid

one five-year study culminating in 1981, reported by The National Academy of Sciences, involving 8,278 Norwegian men, results indicated that the intake of **foods with vitamin A activity** was associated with lower incidence of lung cancer independently of cigarette smoking. This result was extended to women as well as men in the 11-year follow up of the study and in hospital-based case-comparison studies in the United States and in England. Researchers in 1981 hypothesized that the relevant dietary exposure was beta-carotene rather than retinol. This was subsequently supported by a 19-year prospective study of 1,954 middle-aged men in Chicago and population-based case-comparison studies in New Jersey, Hawaii and New Mexico. Two other studies—a 10-year prospective study of 265,118 adults in Japan and a hospital-based case-comparison study of Chinese in Singapore—indicated that lung cancer risk was inversely associated with the frequency of eating green and yellow vegetables.[68]

Carotenes

One of the most notable **components of** vitamin A are carotenes, a group of highly colored plant compounds, some of which can be converted into vitamin A in the intestinal wall and liver, as the body requires. Carotenes are also referred to as *carotenoids*. Beta carotene is the best known of the carotenes, as it offers high pro-vitamin A activity and is abundant in many foods. Other carotenoids include **lutein, zeaxanthin, beta cryptoxanthin, lycopene and alpha carotene.** Carotenoids interact with each other during intestinal absorption, metabolism, and clearance from the body. Because the carotenoids are fat-soluble, they are found in fatty tissues in the body and are transported in blood by lipoproteins.

A 1998 study from Sweden of 124 men and women with lung cancer and 235 people without the disease measured the efficacy of a fruit-and-vegetable

---

[68] *Diet & Health, Implications for Reducing Chronic Disease Risk,* National Research Council, National Academy of Sciences, 1989, page 313.

diet. Findings showed that the risk of lung cancer was 30 percent lower in those with high vegetable intake and 40 percent lower in those consuming "a lot of non-citrus fruits." Results of the study showed that carrots reduced the risk of lung cancer. Researchers speculate that the high beta carotene content in these foods may be the key to lung cancer prevention.[69]

Another Swedish study also reported on the efficacy of foods (not isolated supplements) containing beta carotene with similar optimistic results. The findings were that high beta carotene diets lower breast cancer risk. Of 644 women in this study, 273 had been diagnosed with breast cancer. The women were asked to recall details about their diets throughout their lives. Those reporting diets rich in beta carotene foods for 20 years or more were found to be in the lower risk category than women whose diets included beta carotene only in more recent years, or whose diets were traditionally low in beta carotene foods.[70]

Diets high in fruits and vegetables, with beta carotene under study by a team of Dutch researchers in the late 1990s, show a correlation with reduced risk of heart attack. As part of a four-year Rotterdam study, researchers followed the dietary and medical histories of 4,802 people aged from 55 to 95. Out of 124 of the participants who had heart attacks during this period, analysis showed that those with the highest daily intakes of beta carotene had a 45 percent lower risk of heart attack, compared to people consuming the lowest amount of beta carotene.[71]

As another component of the vitamin A carotenoid complex, **lycopene** has also been studied in its original food form. Lycopene is the carotenoid which gives tomatoes their red color and is one of the major carotenoids in the diet of North Americans and Europeans. It is found in high concentration in the testes, adrenal gland and prostate. Levels of lycopene seem to decrease with age. Several studies suggest that dietary lycopene may help

---

[69] *International Journal of Cancer* 1998;78:430-6.
[70] *Epidemiology* 1999;10:49-53
[71] *American Journal of Clinical Nutrition* 1999; 69:261-6.

prevent cardiovascular disease and cancers of the prostate, pancreas and gastrointestinal tract. According to the results of a 1997 study conducted in Germany, lycopene from tomato paste is more bio-available than lycopene from fresh tomatoes. In a study published in 1995, researchers at Harvard Medical School assessed the links between diet during a one-year period and prostate cancer in almost 48,000 men taking part in the Health Professionals Follow-up Study. They found that men who ate more foods high in lycopene, such as tomatoes, pizza and tomato sauce, were less likely to be at risk of prostate cancer.[72]

In consideration of the entire carotenoid complex, data from the Third National Health and Nutrition Examination Survey suggest prevention against diabetes is also a benefit of diets replete with vitamin A foods. "Researchers from the Centers for Disease Control and Prevention in Atlanta, Georgia, examined concentrations of alpha carotene, beta carotene, cryptoxanthin, lutein/zeaxanthin, and lycopene in 1,010 people (aged from 40 to 74) with normal glucose tolerance. These were compared with those from 277 people with impaired glucose tolerance and 148 people with newly diagnosed diabetes. The results showed that beta carotene and lycopene concentrations were highest in those with normal glucose tolerance, lower in those with impaired glucose tolerance and even lower in people with newly diagnosed diabetes. These results add weight to the evidence that chemicals in fruit and vegetables reduce the risk of developing diabetes.[73]

Problems With Isolated &
Synthetic Vitamin A Supplementation

As mentioned, vitamin A is really a group of compounds (e.g., retinol, retinoids, carotenoids, vitamin A_1 and A_2, etc.) which work synergistically

---

[72] Reavley, 1999, re: *Journal of the National Cancer Institute 1999; 91: 317-331*
[73] Reavley, 1999, re: *American Journal of Epidemiology 1999; 149: 168-76*

with one another in addition to working as cofactors with other nutrients and substances (e.g., iron, bile, etc.). For example, carotenoids need bile acids for absorption and unless they are converted to vitamin A in the wall of the small intestine, they may be absorbed unchanged. Conversion appears to depend on several factors, including protein, thyroid hormone action, zinc and vitamin C. Around 40 to 60 percent of dietary beta carotene is absorbed, although this appears to be reduced in the presence of low stomach acid.[74]

Fractionated and synthetic vitamin A supplements are sold as beta carotene, vitamin A, vitamin A palmitate and synthetic vitamin A derivative drugs including retinoids, and others. Typical of synthetic and even so-called "natural" (but actually really isolated by means of processing) vitamins, vitamin A and vitamin A-related supplements have been reported to create several adverse reactions. When a vitamin is not a part of the original food complex, the chances for toxicity and side effects become possible. Moreover, even by taking a host of vitamin A fractions in an effort to offer "all" of the parts of the vitamin, the entire food complex is never totally recombined and never offers the rest of the synergists and cofactors provided in nature.

> "As vitamin A is fat soluble and can be stored in the liver for long periods of time, it has a high potential for toxicity. The first sign of vitamin A overdose is usually headache, followed by chapped lips, dry skin, fatigue, emotional instability and bone and joint pain. There may also be hair loss, vertigo, vision problems, poor appetite, loss of weight, vomiting, liver damage and amenorrhea (cessation of menstrual periods). Individual tolerance to vitamin A varies widely and these effects can occur at doses over 7,500 mcg RE (25,000 IU) although in most adults signs of toxicity occur with single doses over 75,000 mcg RE

---

[74] Reavley, 1998

(250,000 IU) or smaller doses of 15,000 mcg RE (50,000 IU) taken for long periods. It is recommended that regular daily intake of vitamin A does not exceed 7,500 mcg RE (25 000 IU) for adults and 3,000 mcg RE (10,000 IU) in children.

Pregnant women who take above 3,000 mcg RE (10 000 IU) per day have a greater chance of giving birth to malformed babies. Vitamin A acne cream has been known to cause birth deformities and is now available only on prescription."[75]

Additional research shows...

"In a study published in 1995, researchers at Boston University School of Medicine assessed the links between vitamin A from food and supplements in 22,748 women who were pregnant between October 1984 and June 1987. Women who consumed more than 4,500 mcg RE (15,000 IU) of pre-formed vitamin A per day from food and supplements were over three times more likely to have a baby with a birth defect than women who consumed 1,500 mcg RE (5,000 IU) or less per day. For vitamin A from supplements alone, women who consumed more than 3,000 mcg RE (10,000 IU) per day had almost five times the risk of birth defects than women who consumed less than 1,500 mcg RE (5,000 IU) per day. The increased frequency of defects was concentrated among the babies born to women who had consumed high levels of vitamin A before the seventh week of pregnancy. The researchers estimated that among the babies born to women who took more than 3,000 mcg RE (10,000 IU) of pre-formed vitamin A per day in the form of supplements, about one infant in 57 had a malformation attributable to the supplement.[76]

[75] Mills JL; Simpson JL; Cunningham GC; Conley MR; Rhoads GG. Vitamin A and birth defects. *Am J Obstet Gynecol*, 1997 Jul, 177:1, 31-6
[76] ibid.

"Overdose is reasonably common with as many as 5 percent of people taking vitamin A suffering from the toxicity symptoms. Stopping the large doses usually reverses the symptoms with no lasting damage, although in children damage can be permanent."[77]

"Caution needs to be taken when increasing the intake of any of the lipid soluble vitamins. Excess accumulation of vitamin A in the liver can lead to toxicity which manifests as bone pain, hepatosplenomegaly [enlargement of the liver and spleen], nausea and diarrhea."[78]

A study by Swedish researchers illustrates the possibility of toxic effects of synthetic vitamin A intake and its association with reduced bone density and increased risk of bone fractures and osteoporosis:

"In the first part of the study, researchers measured the bone density of 175 women, aged from 28 to 74. The women were asked to record everything they ate over a typical week and the vitamin A content was calculated. The results showed that in women whose vitamin A intake was more than 1500 mcg per day, bone density was 6 to 14 percent lower than women whose intake was less than 500 mcg per day. In another part of the study, the researchers compared the vitamin A content of the diets of 247 women who had suffered hip fractures with that of 873 women who had not suffered fractures. They found that women whose intake was over 1500 mcg per day had double the risk of fracture compared to women whose intake was less than 500 mcg per day."[79]

Although researchers in the field of nutrition advocate foods containing the carotenoid complex, supplements containing isolated beta carotene may, on the other hand, be deleterious. One study in particular showed

---

[77] Reavley

[78] King

[79] ibid 1998; re: *Annals of Internal Medicine* 1998; 129:770-778

that high doses of beta carotene supplements actually increased lung cancer risk in animal subjects. An animal study has shown that high doses of beta carotene supplements may increase the risk of precancerous changes in lung tissue. The changes were even more pronounced when the animals were exposed to cigarette smoke. For six months, researchers at Tufts University in Boston fed ferrets either a normal diet or a diet supplemented with high doses (equivalent to 30 mg per day in an adult) of beta carotene. Some of the animals were exposed to high doses of cigarette smoke. Examination showed that all of the ferrets receiving high dose supplements had precancerous lesions on lung tissue. This response seemed to be enhanced by exposure to tobacco smoke. Ferrets in the high dose group also had low levels of retinoic acid in their lungs, a form of vitamin A thought to protect against lung cancer.[80] This study tells us that we should:

1. Beware of the effects of isolated beta carotene supplements, and
2. Not allow laboratory animals to smoke.

The concern over the use of beta carotene and vitamin A as isolated and synthetic supplements continues among researchers. Such concern recently led to the early termination of a large scale study on the effects of beta carotene and vitamin A on lung cancer and cardiovascular disease (reported in the *New England Journal of Medicine*):

> A major trial looking into the effects of beta carotene on cancer and cardiovascular disease has been stopped before completion, as results have shown an increased risk of lung cancer and heart disease in those taking beta carotene supplements.
>
> The Beta Carotene and Retinol Efficacy Trial (CARET) was set up to examine the effects of a combination of beta carotene and vitamin A on the incidence of lung cancer in those who were at higher risk of the disease. Over 18,000 smokers, former smokers

---

[80] *Journal of the National Cancer Institute*, 1999; 91:7-8; 60-66.

and workers exposed to asbestos were involved in the trial. The active treatment group received 30mg of beta carotene and 25,000 IU of vitamin A per day and the others received a placebo. The researchers found an increased risk of lung cancer in the group that was receiving beta carotene and vitamin A and stopped the trial 21 months earlier than planned. Follow up will continue for another five years.[81]

In the "CARET"study discussed above, the *Journal of the National Cancer Institute* reported that "Further analysis of data…suggests that the supplements may be harmful in those drinkers and heavy smokers. Those who smoked more than twenty cigarettes a day and drank above average levels of alcohol were found to be adversely affected by the beta carotene supplements."[82] Former smokers were not adversely affected. These results are corroborated by the results of the Alpha Tocopherol Beta Carotene Prevention Trial (ATBC) which was conducted in Finland. There are a number of possible explanations for the adverse effects of beta carotene supplements found in these studies and for the failure of supplements to show the protective effects suggested by epidemiological studies, to wit:

"Beta carotene is susceptible to oxidative damage from alcohol and the gases in cigarette smoke which may lead to the formation of harmful by-products. Beta carotene may be dependent on protection from other antioxidants, such as vitamins C and E to exert protective effects. An individual's total dietary intake of antioxidants may therefore need to be considered when assessing protection by beta carotene.

Beta carotene exists in over 270 possible forms and some research suggests that the specific form chosen for use in these

[81] *Vitamin News*, July 1996, re: *New England Journal of Medicine*, Volume 334, No 18.
[82] *Journal of the National Cancer Institute* 1996; 88.

clinical trials was not the most active agent and that a mixture of various forms of beta carotene, **such as that which occurs naturally, has the most beneficial effect.** It is also possible that the large dose of one particular form of beta carotene competed with other, possibly more beneficial forms at vital sites in the body.

The results of these trials point to the importance of **considering total diet and a balanced mixture of nutrients** when studying protection against cancer risk. High blood levels of carotene seem to predict lower risk and these high blood levels of beta carotene may be accompanied by high levels of other carotenoids which may also play a vital part in cancer protection. Both the ATBC and CARET studies found that those with higher blood beta carotene levels on entering the trials had a lower risk of lung cancer.[83]

Reported in the *New England Journal of Medicine* were the results of a study on beta carotene **supplements** and their lack of effect on the incidence of cancer and heart disease. Although, as stated, many studies indicate that a diet rich in fruits and vegetables seems to protect against cancer and heart attacks (among other diseases), with beta carotene as well as other nutrient complexes (including antioxidants) providing the protection, evidence indicates that isolated beta carotene supplementation fails to offer what whole food complexes provide. "There have been a small number of studies which have found beta carotene to have no protective effect, but it was felt that a larger study over a longer period of time was necessary to fully investigate the disease prevention possibilities. The Physicians Health Study in the United States is one such major project. In this study 22,000 male doctors were given 50 mg of beta

---

[83] ibid.

carotene or placebo every other day for an average of 12 years. The study found that the beta carotene supplements produced neither benefit nor harm in the doctors that were taking them as they did not significantly protect against heart disease or cancer."[84]

The key discovery here is in the recognition by researchers that there is much more to the body's nutrient requirements than can be addressed by isolated substances alone. There is no question that beta carotene is a health-promoting part of foods, yet in various instances it is of questionable value (and possibly harmful) as a fractionated supplement.

---

[84] *New England Journal of Medicine*, Volume 334, No 18.

Vitamin B Complex
& Synergistic Composition

The vitamin B complex is perhaps one of the most overlooked nutrient groups which, when lacking in the diet, leads to deficiencies at the root of countless so-called diseases and "vague" symptoms. In the case of B deficiency, nearly every cell in the body is affected. "The reactions by which B vitamins facilitate energy release take place in every cell, and no cell can do its work without energy...Among the symptoms of B vitamin deficiencies are nausea, severe exhaustion, irritability, depression, forgetfulness, loss of appetite and weight, pain in muscles, impairment of the immune response, loss of control of the limbs, abnormal heart action, severe skin problems, teary or bloodshot eyes, and many more [irregular heartbeat, enlarged heart, blood cell damage, cracks in the sides of the mouth, digestive disturbances, swollen tongue, brain damage, chronic fatigue, paranoia, attention deficit]. Because cell renewal depends on energy, protein and DNA/RNA availability, and because all of these depend on the B vitamins, tissues in which the cells' life spans are shortest are most readily damaged by B vitamin deficiency."[85]

Jack Cooperman, Ph.D., New York Medical College (director of nutrition) states that "It takes only a few weeks for the [vitamin] B levels in your

---

[85] Hamilton, page 206.

blood to drop. This increases the risk of a subclinical deficiency, which can occur after active forms of the B vitamins in the cells decrease."[86]

Despite the subclinical, symptomatic evidence of vitamin B deficiency, as of this writing, the standard expression of the scientific community is that vitamin B deficiency is rare in this day and age of mass enrichment and fortification of foods. However, because enrichment is performed with synthetic vitamins, it appears that such synthetic use of vitamin B fails to provide the body with what it needs to achieve optimal health. Food-based vitamin B, on the other hand, is found along with important cofactors inherent in the whole food provide constituents that enable B vitamins to be metabolized and used as nutrients for a plethora of functions.

"The B vitamins are often found together in food and were first thought to be a single substance needed to produce energy from food. They are now known to be eight individual nutrients with separate coenzyme functions required for various steps in the metabolism of carbohydrate, protein and fat. The B vitamins also interact; some are needed to convert others into their active coenzyme forms, and a deficiency of any one can interfere with energy metabolism and cause some common deficiency symptoms. For example, depression and weakness may result from a deficiency of one or more of the B vitamins."[87]

Joan Priestly, M.D. and health editor Carolyn Reuben concur, writing, "if you take a disproportionately large dose of one B vitamin, after a few weeks the body will begin to complain with myriad distress symptoms. It needs the other Bs to use any one of them effectively."[88]

"In academic discussions of the vitamins, clearly different deficiency symptoms are given for each one. Actually such clear-cut symptoms are found only in laboratory animals that have been fed contrived diets that lack just one ingredient. In real life, a deficiency of any one B vitamin seldom

---

[86] Faelten, Sharon, Ed., *The Complete Book of Vitamins and Minerals*, Rodale Press, Inc., New Jersey, 1988, page 92.

[87] Smolin, page 280.

[88] Reuben, page 135.

shows up by mixtures of nutrients. Still the deficiency of one B vitamin may appear predominant in a cluster of deficiencies, and often, if it is corrected by giving **wholesome food rather than single supplements**, the subtler deficiencies will be corrected along with it."[89]

Thiamin

Thiamin is the name given to vitamin B_1 which is widely distributed in many foods and is a water-soluble component of the B complex of vitamins. First isolated in 1926, thiamin is present in yeast, milk, meat, nuts, beans, green vegetables, sweet corn, egg yolk, liver, corn meal and brown rice. Fresh yeast and wheat germ offer the highest concentrations of thiamin. Vegetables contain very little vitamin B_1.

Thiamin, found in blood plasma and cerebrospinal fluid in the free state, is a water-soluble substance, consisting of thiazole and pyrimidine rings joined by a methylene bridge, with both moieties (portions) needed for full biologic action. Thiamin pyrophosphate (TPP) is the active form of thiamin. Reducing very involved biochemical descriptions into simplified terms, thiamin is involved in the production of energy from carbohydrates, converting sugars to even simpler substances, the transmission of nerve impulses, the breaking down of sugars into simpler compounds, the making of fatty acids, acetylcholine production, and the formation of nucleic acids. TPP has been implicated also in sodium movement and impulse initiation in neuronal membranes.[90] During a deficiency of thiamin, pyruvic acid accumulates in the blood and carbohydrates is not properly metabolized.[91]

---

[89] Hamilton, page 208.

[90] American Society of Nutritional Sciences: Tanphaichitr, V. (1994) *Thiamin. In: Modern Nutrition in Health and Disease* (Shils, M.E., Olson, J.A., & Shike, M., eds.), 8th ed., vol. 1, pp. 359-365. Lea & Febiger, Philadelphia, PA, and Tan, G.H., Farnell, G.F., Hensrud, D.D. & Litin, S.C. (1994) Acute Wernicke's encephalopathy attributable to pure dietary thiamine deficiency. *Mayo. Clin. Proc.* 69: 849-850.

[91] ibid, page 281.

Thus, thiamin is particularly important in brain and nerve tissue, which must use glucose as an energy source. Due to thiamin's effect on nervous system activity, a deficiency may lead to poor coordination and nervous tingling in the arms and legs. Thiamin is also needed for the synthesis of the neurotransmitter acetylcholine; and the metabolism of alcohol.[92] As a coenzyme needed for the synthesis of sugars such as ribose, thiamin is necessary to produce the nucleotides of nucleic acids, including RNA.

Chemistry textbooks note that thiamine has been crystallized as a hydrochloride (converted from its natural nutrient state) and that it is soluble in water and also in alcohol up to 70 percent. Thiamine is stable in acid solution but is destroyed in alkaline and neutral solutions. It is also somewhat stable in low heat and can be sterilized for 30 minutes at 120 degrees (C) without appreciable loss in activity. The crystallized version of the vitamin, *thiamine hydrochloride*, is a salt produced by treating thiamine with hydrochloric acid and is more soluble than thiamine itself, which is why it is used as an isolated vitamin B_1 supplement.[93]

As with any nutrient, the amount of thiamin needed in the daily diet depends on the needs of each individual, as well as on many other factors. The body needs more thiamin in the event of a fever, increased muscular activity, hyperthyroidism, pregnancy and lactation. The thiamin requirement of the body also increases during a diet high in carbohydrates, and decreases with a diet high in fat and protein. For these reasons, and because of thiamin's interaction with other nutrients, as well as the rest of the vitamin B complex, thiamin is best ingested in whole foods.

There is speculation that diets excessively high in foods containing *thiaminases* (enzymes that degrade thiamin) may lead to depletion of vitamin B_1. Such foods include coffee, certain types of raw fish, tea, betel nuts, blueberries and red cabbage.[94]

---

[92] ibid, page 282.

[93] Sackheim, page 434

[94] Smolin, page 281, Re: *Annual New York Academy of Sciences*, 378:123-136, 1982.

Alcoholics are also likely to suffer from thiamin deficiency because thiamin is needed for alcohol metabolism; and alcohol decreases the absorption of thaimin. Tobacco smokers are also at risk of thiamin deficiency, as well as patients with chronic fevers and kidney failure.

Vitamin B₁ deficiency initially leads to loss of appetite, failure of growth and loss of weight, and if left unchecked, leads to a disease known as beriberi (in animals this disease is referred to as *polyneuritis*). Beriberi was at first thought to occur only in the Orient where fish and polished rice (both lacking vitamin B₁) are mainstays of the diet. In most of the world, modern food processing removes vitamin B₁ along with other B vitamins and nutrients. The thiamin-containing portions of plant foods (bran, germ, etc.) are stripped away mainly because of their oil-containing constituents, which are prone to spoiling, and are a liability to food producers banking on shelf life.

Like so many other instances of vitamin deficiency, scientists at first expended much energy and time looking for a microbial causation for beriberi before realizing that it was not caused by an environmental pathogen or toxin. Prior to the year 1900, a prison physician in the East Indies discovered that beriberi could be cured with proper diet. He noticed that chickens at the prison developed a stiffness and weakness similar to that of prisoners who had beriberi. The chickens were being fed scraps from the polished rice diet of the prisoners. When fed rice bran, the paralysis of the chickens was cured. Upon this discovery, prisoners who were subsequently fed discarded rice bran (full of nutrients) also were cured.[95]

Beriberi leads to a degeneration of certain nerves leading to the muscles. Pressure applied along these nerves causes pain, and eventually the muscles served by these nerves begin to atrophy from disuse. This leads several modern-day researchers to conclude that painful fibromyalgia is

---

[95] Hamilton, page 208

primarily a deficiency of vitamin B_1, and the rest of the entire B complex, as well as certain other supportive and synergistic nutrients. Without thiamin, beriberi may be fatal, as the heart enlarges and death from heart failure ensues.

Malaria victims are equally in need of thiamin, as scientists in the United Kingdom and Thailand recently suggested. Researchers compared the levels of thiamin in the blood of 77 patients with malaria with those of 50 people who had no trace of the malaria parasite in their blood. The results showed that "12 of the 23 patients with severe malaria and 10 of the 54 patients with uncomplicated malaria tested positive for thiamin deficiency." None of the control patients had deficiency symptoms. Thiamin deficiency was especially pronounced in those who died from the disease.[96]

Thiamin is absorbed primarily through the wall of the duodenum and is transported by the blood to body cells. Only small amounts are stored in the tissues, and excesses are excreted in the urine.

In blood, thiamin is present in erythrocytes (red blood cells) as well as in plasma where it is bound largely to albumin (a protein).

Thiamin deficiencies "consist of central nervous manifestations, including mystagmus, ophthalmoplegia, ataxia and memory deficit usually termed collectively as Wernicke's syndrome. This may merge into more extensive mental confusion with confabulation [imagined memory], usually called *Korsakoff's psychosis*. Another manifestation of thiamin deficiency, often in the setting of alcoholism, is peripheral neuropathy...Cardiomegaly and congestive heart failure, with a characteristic high cardiac output presumably related to low peripheral resistance, is seen in thiamin deficiency and is termed cardiac (Shoshin) beriberi. The precise pathogenic mechanisms of these clinical syndromes are still uncertain, but are felt to be reflections of deranged carbohydrate metabolism, likely affecting the decarboxylation pathway. Detection of thiamin deficiency depends on a high

[96] *The Lancet* 1999;353:546-549

index of suspicion (i.e., the syndrome may be seen with poor food intake, prolonged vomiting, intake of thiaminases in some types of fish and not just alcoholism) and the use of confirmatory laboratory tests. These include the measurement of erythrocyte transketolase activity and its enhancement on in vitro addition of thiamin pyrophosphate (TPP effect) and blood thiamin levels. The TPP effect may not be seen with chronic thiamin loss."[97]

As part of the vitamin B complex, thiamin is found in B complex foods such as legumes, yeast, lean pork, etc. Thiamin is destroyed at high temperatures (cooking) and at pH above 8.

Riboflavin

Riboflavin is the name given to vitamin B_2, a widely distributed vitamin known to function in oxidation-reduction reactions. Riboflavin is the precursor for the coenzymes **flavin mononucleotide (FMN)** and **flavin adenine dinucleotide (FAD)**. Enzymes requiring FMN or FAD as cofactors are *flavoproteins*. Several flavoproteins also contain metal ions and are termed *metallo*flavoproteins. Both classes of enzymes are involved in a wide range of redox (oxidation-reduction) reactions, e.g. *succinate dehydrogenase* and *xanthine oxidase*.[98] In conjunction with other B vitamins, riboflavin works to oxidize fat and carbohydrate to carbon dioxide to produce energy. "The complete oxidation of these fuels occurs via the Kreb's Cycle, a sequence of enzyme-catalyzed steps that represents the major energy-yielding pathway of most tissues.[99]

Riboflavin oxidizes toxins and foreign compounds in maintaining the body's defense system. It is also known to support *glutathione reductase*, an enzyme that replenishes glutathione, an important cellular antioxidant. This system represents a major defense against oxidative damage.

---

[97] American Society of Nutritional Sciences: Tanphaichitr, V.
[98] King
[99] Ronzio, page 381.

Riboflavin is also needed for the production of steroid hormones by the adrenal glands. And riboflavin is required for successful reproduction, as evidenced with experimental animals, as well as for healthy skin, eyes and nerve function.

Arguably, researchers have noted that a deficiency in riboflavin does not point to a specific disease. Instead, disease states occur in association with other important B vitamin deficiencies associated with riboflavin deficiency. With this noted, riboflavin deficiency (*ariboflavinosis*) may include fatigue, weakness, delayed wound healing, sore mouth, sore throat, hyperemia, cheilosis (cracks in the corners of the mouth), tongue inflammation (glossitis), blurred vision and light sensitivity, seborrheic dermatitis, corneal vascularization, eczema of face and genitalia and normochromic, normocytic anemia associated with pure red cell hypoplasia (underdevelopment) of the bone marrow.[100, 101] Other symptoms may include seborrhea, angular stomatitis (inflammation of oral mucosa), and photophobia (abnormal visual intolerance of light).

Riboflavin decomposes when exposed to visible light. This characteristic can lead to riboflavin deficiencies in newborns treated for hyperbilirubinemia by phototherapy.[102]

Riboflavin is found in whole foods along with other naturally occurring B vitamins. Riboflavin is extremely light-and heat-sensitive, especially in instances of pasteurization or heating (cooking). Fruits and vegetables contain very little of this B vitamin, yet vegetarians may find it in wheat, mushrooms, yeast, raw milk and cheese products and soybean flour. Meat and dairy products are good sources.

Riboflavin functions as a part of several enzymes and coenzymes known as *flavoproteins* essential for the oxidation of glucose and fatty acids, and for cellular growth. Its absorption seems to be regulated by an active transport system controlling how much riboflavin will be taken in by the intestinal

---

[100] American Society of Nutritional Sciences
[101] ibid
[102] King

mucosa, and it is carried in the blood combined with blood proteins called *albumins*. Excessive amounts of riboflavin are excreted in the urine, and unabsorbed amounts are lost in the feces.[103]

Niacin

Niacin, also known as vitamin B3, or nicotinic acid, is found in plant tissues and is relatively stable in the face of heat, acids and alkalis. After ingestion, niacin is converted by human cells to a physiologically active form called *niacinamide*, and "it is also in this form that the vitamin is present in foods of animal origin."[104]

> "Niacin (nicotinic acid or nicotinamide) is essential in the form of the coenzymes nicotinamide adenine dinucleotide (NAD) and NAD phosphate (NADP) in which the nicotinamide moiety acts as an electron acceptor or hydrogen donor in many biological redox reactions. NAD functions as an electron carrier for intracellular respiration, as well as a codehydrogenase with enzymes involved in the oxidation of fuel molecules. NADP functions as a hydrogen donor in reductive biosyntheses such as in fatty acid and steroid syntheses and, like NAD, as a codehydrogenase...Nicotinic acid and nicotinamide are rapidly absorbed from the stomach or the intestine. Nicotinamide, the major form in the bloodstream, arises from enzymatic hydrolysis of NADP in the intestinal mucosa and liver. It is transported to tissues that synthesize their own NAD as needed. Niacin and NAD are biosynthesized from dietary tryptophan..."[105]

---

[103] Hole, John Jr., *Human Anatomy & Physiology*, William C. Brown Company Publishers, Iowa, 1978, page 471.

[104] ibid

[105] American Society of Nutritional Sciences: Swendseid, M.E., & Jacob, R.A. (1994) Niacin. In: Modern Nutrition in Health and Disease (Shils, M.E., Olson, J.A. & Shike, M., eds.), 8th ed., pp. 376-382. Lea & Febiger, Philadelphia, PA.

Niacin combines with riboflavin (and thiamin) to oxidize foods, allowing the cells to produce adequate amounts of energy in the mitochondria. Niacin and riboflavin are used to form coenzymes and flavoprotein, required during the oxidation of hydrogen to combine with hydrogen atoms after they are removed from pyruvic acid and other substrates.[106] Niacin functions in the mitochondria as part of two coenzymes—coenzyme I (also known as NAD, *nicotinamide adenine dinucleotide*) and coenzyme II (called NADP, *nicotinamide adenine dinucleotide phosphate*) which play essential roles in the oxidation of glucose and in the synthesis of proteins and fats. These coenzymes are needed for the synthesis of sugars used in the production of nucleic acids.[107]

Niacin can be ingested from foods as well as synthesized by human cells from the essential amino acid *tryptophan*. Therefore, physiologists and biochemists state that the need for niacin is related proportionately to the need or presence of tryptophan. "It is believed that 60mg of tryptophan is equivalent to 1mg of niacin, but this equivalence seems to vary from one individual to another."[108] Some niacin may also be synthesized by bacterial action in the intestines and thus become available for use.

As a side note, many natural doctors have been scrambling for tryptophan once the FDA took the supplement off the shelves. Ironically, most "natural" healthcare practitioners forgot that, like any other nutrient, natural tryptophan is to be found in foods. Botanist-researcher, Dr. James Duke, writes: "Since the tryptophan scare, some people have been at loose ends about natural sedatives. With that in mind, I went to my FNF database to see what was my best food or dietary source of tryptophan. What should come out highest but evening primrose seed, with up to 16,000 ppm's on a dry weight basis." Other relatively high sources were (on a zero-moisture dry-weight):

---

[106] Guyton, page 392
[107] Hole, page 471
[108] ibid, page 473

Tryptophan Sources	PPM
Almond	up to 3,500
Amaranth	up to 3,500
Barley	up to 3,000
Butternut	up to 3,000
Cabbage	up to 3,000
Cowpea	up to 3,000
Evening Primrose Seed	up to 16,000
Fenugreek	up to 4,000
Kidney Bean	up to 2,500
Lima Bean	up to 3,000
Mungbean	up to 3,500
Mustard Seed (white)	up to 5,500
Oats	up to 3,000
Pistachio	up to 3,000
Poppy Seed	up to 2,500
Pumpkin Seed	up to 4,500
Sesame	up to 5,000
Spinach	up to 4,500
Sunflower	up to 4,000
Watercress	up to 6,000
Wheat	up to 3,000
Winged Bean	up to 8,000

Niacin deficiency results in discoloration of the skin, which darkens upon exposure to sunlight. This is followed by severe weakness, diarrhea and one or more psychoses. (Niacin deficiency in dogs produces tongue lesions called black tongue). The host of symptoms, as well as digestive tract inflammation and dermatitis, is due to vitamin B_1 deficiency known as *pellagra*. Pellagra comes from the Italian *pelle agra*, meaning "rough skin." Originally, niacin was called nicotinic acid, or "the antipellagra factor."

As with most other nutrients, niacin requires cofactors to function biochemically. Therefore, a deficiency of niacin is usually accompanied by a deficiency in other substances as well.

Physiologist Arthur C. Guyton, M.D. writes: "Deficiency of riboflavin is not as likely to lead to such severe difficulties as deficiency of niacin, because other types of flavoproteins that can perform almost the same functions as the protein derived from riboflavin are present in the body. Nevertheless, riboflavin deficiency, when occurring along with deficiencies of niacin or thiamine, can greatly intensify the symptoms observed in pellagra or beriberi. A common result of riboflavin deficiency alone is cracking at the angles of the mouth, called *cheilosis*."[109]

Niacin, along with synergistic vitamins (especially of the B complex), is found in asparagus, yeast, barley, legumes, soybeans, dried beans, beef, chicken, collards, corn, lamb, liver, some fish (mackerel, salmon), wheat and pork. Historically speaking, deficiencies of niacin have presented in diets high in corn and corn products combined with pork fat (especially noticeable in the pre-Civil War South in the poor and limited diets of African slaves, and even up to the early 1900s in the rural southern states) which are very low in niacin and deficient in tryptophan (and high protein foods). Both niacin and tryptophan occur in liver, lean meats, poultry, peanut butter and legumes. Milk, a poor source of niacin, is a good source of tryptophan.

Generally, there is a slightly greater need for niacin in the diet by pregnant and lactating mothers and adolescents.

The isolated supplement form of niacin is relatively unpredictable from individual to individual. Some report mild flushing (redness) and tingling of the skin, while others have experienced burning, extreme flushing and even severe intestinal cramping with nausea and headache.

---

[109] ibid, page 393

Researcher Dr. Ralph Golan writes, "Niacinamide has the potential in large doses to cause a temporary inflammation of the liver, which may result in nausea, abdominal discomfort and other symptoms. Stopping it and then resuming at a lower dose usually resolves the trouble. It is important in long term users to have liver enzyme levels checked periodically with a simple blood test. Those with current liver disease should not take high dose niacinamide without the supervision of a health care professional, and some, possibly, should not take it at all."[110]

As in the use of other fractionated vitamins, the results are pharmacological with possible accompanying biochemical imbalance that may or may not become immediately and clinically evident. One study showed that "nicotinic acid (but not nicotinamide) when administered in pharmacological doses of 2—4 g/day lowers plasma cholesterol levels and has been shown to be a useful therapeutic for hypercholesterolemia. The major action of nicotinic acid in this capacity is a reduction in fatty acid mobilization from adipose tissue. **Although nicotinic acid therapy lowers blood cholesterol it also causes a depletion of glycogen stores and fat reserves** in skeletal and cardiac muscle. Additionally, there is an elevation in blood glucose and uric acid production. For these reasons nicotinic acid therapy is not recommended for diabetics or persons who suffer from gout."[111] In the opinion of naturalists, this is yet another example of the unpredictability of using a isolated vitamin substances upon biochemical systems, directly or indirectly associated with those which are attempted to be therapeutically addressed.

Pyridoxine

Originally known as the "rat antidermatitis factor," vitamin B6 is made up of pyridoxine, pyridoxal and pyridoxamine. Since these compounds are

---

[110] Golan, Dr. Ralph, *Finding Options for Easing Osteoarthritis*, OnHealth Network Company online; December 02, 1999
[111] King

readily interconvertible, the accepted term for vitamin B$_6$ is pyridoxine. Pyridoxine is found in yeast, liver, egg yolk, and the germ of various grains and seeds. It is also found to a limited extent in milk and leafy vegetables.[112]

The American Society for Nutritional Sciences explains:

> About 70-80 percent of the vitamin B$_6$ in the body is located in muscle bound to glycogen phosphorylase, an enzyme involved in releasing glucose from glycogen. About 10 percent is located in the liver. The remainder is distributed among the other tissues.
>
> Vitamin B$_6$ is one of the most versatile enzyme cofactors. It is involved in breaking more types of chemical bonds than most cofactors. It is listed in Enzyme Nomenclature as a component of approximately 120 enzymes including at least one entry in 5 of the 6 major enzyme classes. Pyridoxal phosphate is a cofactor in the metabolism of amino acids and neurotransmitters and in the breakdown of glycogen. Pyridoxal phosphate can bind to steroid hormone receptors and may have a role in regulating steroid hormone action. Pyridoxal phosphate plays a role in the immune system; thus adequate intake is important. 4-pyridoxic acid is the major excretory product.
>
> Alterations in the function of the nervous system evidenced by electroencephalography are among the earliest symptoms of vitamin B$_6$ deficiency. Severe deficiency may produce seizures, dermatitis, glossitis, cheilosis, angular stomatitis and anemia. Frank deficiencies are rare, but subclinical deficiencies may exist, especially in women and the elderly.[113]

112 Sackheim, page 438.
113 American Society for Nutritional Sciences: Leklem, J.E. (1990) Vitamin B6. In: *Handbook of Vitamins* (I.J. Machlin, ed.), 2nd ed. pp. 341-392. Marcel Dekker, New York, N.Y. and Raiten, D.J. ed. (1995) *Vitamin B6 Metabolism in Pregnancy, Lactation, and Infancy.* CRC Press, Boca Raton, FL.

Folic Acid/Folate

Folic acid (folate) is also known as *folacin* and *pteroylglutamic acid* (PGA) (pronounced *tare-oil-glue-TAM-ick*) as well as vitamin M. Biochemistry teaches that PGA is only one of several related compounds in the folic acid group. Others are pteroic acid, pterolytriglutamic acid, and pteroylheptaglutamic acid.[114] Folate is a B vitamin and its coenzyme (a small molecule that works with an enzyme to promote the enzyme's activity) forms are DHF (dihydrofolate) and THF (terahydrofolate). THF is part of an enzyme complex responsible for handling one-carbon units arising during metabolism; an action critical to processes such as synthesis of the DNA required for rapidly growing cells, including those of the GI tract, blood and all fetal tissues.[115] Folic acid is concerned with the transfer of methyl groups in the formation of such compounds as choline and methionine.

Folic acid is especially important in the formation of red and white blood cells and blood platelets. As a result of folate deficiency anemia takes place. Therefore, pernicious anemia, macrocytic anemia (presence of giant red corpuscles) and sprue are greatly benefited by the addition of folic acid to the diet.

The body receives folate mostly from foods in the bound form; that is, folate combined with a string of amino acids (glutamic acid), known as polyglutamate. "The intestine prefers to absorb the 'free' folate form—folate with only one glutamate attached (the monoglutamate form), sometimes with a methyl (CH3) group attached, also. Enzymes on the surfaces of the intestinal cells hydrolyze the polyglutamate and then may attach the methyl group; special transport systems take up the monoglutamate either with or without a methyl group; and both travel freely in the blood."[116]

The liver takes both of the above forms and handles them differently. Monoglutamate, in the liver, is combined with additional glutamates and

114 Sackheim, page 441.
115 Hamilton, page 209.
116 ibid.

converted into polyglutamate to be stored. The methyl form of folate is secreted by the liver in bile and then delivered into the gallbladder where it returns once again to the intestines. "Should the methyl folate be needed within the body, the methyl group would have to be removed—and the enzyme that removes it requires another B vitamin as a coenzyme; vitamin B_{12}..."[117]

Cells of organs other than the liver also absorb the monoglutamate form of folate and then add glutamates to keep the monoglutamate from leaving. To release it, these various cells hydrolyze the monoglutamate so that it may be used elsewhere. The complex system of converting, using, storing and releasing folate is dependent on many biochemical processes. For instance, a healthy intestinal tract is needed for reabsorption of folate. A faulty GI tract may result in the loss of folate and folate deficiency. Alcohol abuse is one such example of how the GI tract can be impaired.

Folate enzymes are active in cell multiplication. Thus, because cells lining the GI tract are among the most rapidly renewed cells in the body, any impediment to making new cells results in rapid deterioration. This leads not only to folate loss, but also the inability to absorb other nutrients.

Sources of folate include leafy green vegetables, legumes, seeds, yeast, kidney, cauliflower and liver. However, as has been stated, even with an intake of folate-rich foods, without a healthy GI tract, folate deficiency symptoms and disease may be present. Such deficiencies have been seen in alcoholism, empty calorie diets, infants fed on goats' milk (low in folate), and in various diseases in which cell multiplication is required to speed up—cancer, multiple pregnancies, skin-destroying diseases (chicken pox, measles), burns, blood loss, etc.

A deficiency in folate may result in the impairment of cell division and protein synthesis—"processes critical to growing tissues. In a folate deficiency, the replacement of red blood cells and GI tract cells falters.

---

[117] ibid.

Not surprisingly then, two of the first symptoms of a deficiency of folate are a type of anemia and GI tract deterioration."[118]

Folic acid, in a nonfood, isolated supplement form has been reported to possibly mask the effects of vitamin B12 deficiency, which is especially noted among vegetarians. The risk of anemia and nerve damage has been suspected by the authors of a review in a 1998 edition of *Archives of Internal Medicine:* "While it is rare, there have been cases where folic acid has masked vitamin B_{12} deficiency and led to seizures in patients with epilepsy, zinc deficiency and incidence of cancer and malaria…The author of the study, Dr. Norman Campbell from the University of Calgary in Canada suggests that if folic acid intake is increased the lowest dose that would ensure benefit should be used."[119]

Cobalamin (Vitamin B12)

"The distinction between vitamin B_{12} and folate was blurry until the middle of this century. Their roles intertwine, but each serves a specific function that the other cannot perform. They share a special relationship: vitamin B_{12} assists the enzyme that removes the methyl group from methyl folate, thus regenerating the folate coenzyme THF. Its action is evident whenever cells are rapidly dividing. Vitamin B_{12} also maintains the sheath that surrounds and protects nerve fibers and promotes their normal growth. In addition to these two primary roles of vitamin B_{12}, bone cell activity and metabolism seem to depend on its presence."[120]

Vitamin B_{12} (named *cobalamin* because this vitamin contains the element cobalt at 4.35 percent) is found in animal food sources, including organ meats (liver and kidney), bivalve mollusks (clams and oysters) and, in lesser amounts, in poultry, egg yolks, fermented cheeses and dry milk.

---

[118] ibid.
[119] *Vitamin News*, Sept. 1996; re: *Archives of Internal Medicine*, 1996: 156
[120] ibid, page 212.

Algae such as nori and spirulina contain vitamin B_{12} analogs that are argued to be biologically inactive in humans. Animal and fish muscle contain very small amounts of vitamin B_{12}.

Vitamin B_{12} is stored in the liver and is a co-factor for two coenzymes. Methyl-cobalamin catalyzes methyl group transfer from a folic acid co-factor to form methionine. The unmethylated folate co-factor then participates in single carbon reactions for nucleic acid synthesis. Thus some symptoms of vitamin B_{12} and folic acid deficiencies are similar. The B_{12} coenzyme deoxyadenosylcobalamin catalyzes amino and fatty acid breakdown.[121]

Vitamin B_{12} deficiency, as a disease-state, is referred to as *pernicious anemia* because vitamin B_{12}, along with folic acid, are needed by the bone marrow to form red blood cells. Folic acid and vitamin B_{12} are also needed in all the other tissues of the body for adequate growth. When vitamin B_{12} deficiency occurs, the red blood cells released into the blood are few in number, and those that are released are usually larger than normal, poorly formed, and very fragile. The result is a severe anemia (pernicious anemia).[122] Vitamin B_{12} deficiency does not necessarily mean that there is a deficiency in the ingestion of vitamin B_{12}. Because the origin of pernicious anemia may be also attributed to a lack of the intrinsic factor in the gastric juice. This may be the result of gastrectomy, a severe thyroid problem or atrophy of the gastric mucosa.[123]

Intrinsic factor mediates the absorption of vitamin B_{12} at various receptor sites in the ileum. In the elderly, *atrophic gastritis* is commonly associated with the inability to absorb vitamin B_{12} which then is secreted in the bile and subsequently reabsorbed. In essence, then, not only does a lack of vitamin B_{12} lead to pernicious anemia, but also pernicious anemia leads to further vitamin B_{12} deficiency. Due to the cycle wherein the vitamin is

---

[121] ibid.

[122] Guyton, page 393.

[123] Mosby Medical Encylopedia, Signet, Missouri, 1996. page 426.

absorbed, redistributed then reabsorbed, some researchers claim that deficiency symptoms may take 20 years to develop from low vitamin B_{12} intake, particularly as related to strict vegetarians. In malabsorption, however, deficiency occurs "in months or a few years because absorption from both the diet and enterohepatic circulation is impaired."[124]

Guyton writes: "On studying the bone marrow one finds that the new red cells being formed have abnormal structures, for which reason it is believed that B_{12} and folic acid are necessary for the formation of the structural elements of the cells. However, lack of these vitamins does not affect the formation of hemoglobin."[125]

Guyton also writes that red blood cells are affected more than other bodily cells in the instances of vitamin B_{12} and folic acid deficiency probably because these cells are produced faster than other cells.[126]

Stages of vitamin B_{12} deficiencies range from affecting the red blood cells to possible irreversible demyelination of the spinal cord, brain and optic and peripheral nerves, producing peripheral neuropathy progressing to subacute combined degeneration. Early symptoms may include dementia, poor attention span and depression.

Recent research (as of 1999) shows that vitamin B_{12} deficiency "may increase the risk of neural tube defects in pregnant women with a high risk of this condition. Vitamin B_{12} deficiency may be common in AIDS and also in developing countries, probably due to malabsorption combined with low intakes."[127]

According to one study at the University of Georgia (1999), low levels of B vitamins were found to cause hearing impairment. More specifically, in a

[124] American Society of Nutritional Sciences: Herbert, V. (1996) Vitamin B-12. In: *Present Knowledge in Nutrition* (Filer, L.J. & Ziegler, E., eds.), 7th ed., pp. 191-205. International Life Sciences Institute Press, Washington, DC ; and Allen, L.H. & Casterline, J. (1994) Vitamin B-12 deficiency in the elderly: diagnosis and requirements. *Am. J. Clin. Nutr.* 60: 12-14.

[125] ibid.

[126] ibid.

[127] ibid.

small study of 55 healthy women ages 60 to 71, vitamin B_{12} and folate were linked to hearing loss. In this group, women with damaged hearing had 38 percent lower vitamin B_{12} and 31 percent lower red cell folate than women with normal hearing.[128]

Choline

Vitamin B_{12} is involved in the synthesis of some amino acids as well as in choline. Although choline is essential, it is not considered a vitamin because it can be synthesized in the body and is required in greater amounts than are vitamins. A deficiency in choline may lead to such symptoms as fatty liver, hemorrhagic degeneration of the kidneys, cirrhosis, perosis (slipped tendon disease), and more. Choline is a constituent of *lecithin* and *sphingomyelin* (phosopholipids which occur primarily in nervous tissue and generally in membranes) and is important in brain and nervous tissue. Proteins supply amino acids from which choline may be synthesized; and therefore a choline deficiency is less likely to develop in a person on a high protein diet.[129]

---

[128] *American Journal of Clinical Nutrition,* 1999; 69; 564-571.
[129] Sackheim, page 444.

VITAMIN C COMPLEX & SYNERGISTIC COMPOSITION

Perhaps no other vitamin has gained such popularity and promise as vitamin C. Much of this attention has resulted from the work of Nobel Award-winning scientist Linus Pauling and his appraisal of ascorbic acid. Recommending megadoses, Pauling reported the wonders of ascorbic acid—from essential to miraculous. Yet many biochemical researchers make careful note to distinguish between studies of ascorbic acid and that of the entire, food-source vitamin C complex (containing not only ascorbic acid, but many other constituents and cofactors, such as rutin, copper, bioflavonoids, etc.). As vitamin C synergists, bioflavonoids protect vitamin C from destruction in the body by oxidation.[130] The bioflavonoid complex (discussed later) contains citrin, hesperidin, quercitin, and rutin. as well as thousands of others.

Bioflavonoids were once considered vitamins (vitamin P) because they work so closely with vitamin C. It can be argued, therefore, that the importance of bioflavonoids as part of the whole vitamin C complex (and completely absent in the fractionated/synthetic vitamin C supplement pill) cannot be understated. Found in the rind of citrus fruits, bioflavonoids are helpful in the absorption of vitamin C. As part of the vitamin C complex, bioflavonoids have been shown to strengthen capillary walls as well as the walls of smooth muscle tissue and epithelial cells. As such, vitamin C foods

---

[130] Airola, Ph.D., N.D., Paavo, *How to Get Well*, Health Plus Publishers, Sherwood, Oregon, 1974, p. 271.

help with varicose veins, hemorrhages, bruises, incontinence, cataracts and skin tissue repair. Working with the rest of the vitamin C complex, bioflavonoids play an essential role in allowing the body to carry on the function of inflammation and repair.

Gabe Mirkins, M.D. bluntly challenges the long-standing research of Linus Pauling and the vitamin C miracle pill, stating:

The latest research [on vitamin C] shows that Linus Pauling was wrong. A recent report in the Proceedings of the National Academy of Sciences shows that the optimal dose of vitamin C is closer to 200 mg per day, not 4000. Blood levels of vitamin C were first depleted by placing men on a diet that contained fewer than 5 milligrams of vitamin C per day. Then the men continued their vitamin C deficient diet and took vitamin pills ranging from 30 to 2500 mg of vitamin C each day. White blood cells were saturated at 100 mg per day and couldn't take in any more vitamin C and blood fluid was saturated at 200 mg per day. Beyond 100 mg per day, the volunteers excreted huge amounts of vitamin C in their urine showing that their bodies couldn't retain that much. At 1000 mg per day, breakdown products of vitamin C called *oxalates* and those of nucleic acids called *urates*, started to accumulate in the urine. Each can cause kidney stones in susceptible people. Large doses of vitamin C can also cause liver and heart damage in people who have an inherited condition that causes them to take in too much iron.

This study shows that you can get all the vitamin C that you can keep by eating each day, any one of 2 oranges, 2 grapefruits, 2 peppers, 2 kiwi fruits, 2 cups of broccoli or brussels sprouts or drinking 2 glasses of cranberry juice. Besides, you will also meet your needs for other vitamins, minerals, fiber and phytochemicals that are found in all fruits, vegetables, whole grains and beans.[131]

131 Mirkin, M.D., Gabe, citing: Levine, Mark. Proceedings of the National Academy of Sciences. Report #6787 April, 1996.

Some practitioners argue that food complexes of vitamin C achieve NUTRITIVE results, as opposed to only pharmacological (drug-like) effects achieved with the use of synthetic isolated ascorbic acid (made from corn sugar and sold as vitamin C supplements). Indeed, **any vitamin in an isolated form requires at least the presence of certain cofactors for results.** Author Elson M. Haas, M.D. writes, "Overall, it is probably best to take vitamin C as it is found in nature, along with the vitamin P constituents— the bioflavonoids, rutin, and hesperidin. These may have a synergistic influence on the functions of vitamin C…"

Haas writes, "In recent years, the *C* of this much-publicized vitamin has…stood for *C*ontroversy. With Linus Pauling and others claiming that vitamin C has the potential to prevent and treat the common cold, flus, and cancer, all of which plague our society, concern has arisen in the medical establishment about these claims and the megadose requirements needed to achieve the hoped-for results. Some studies suggest that these claims have some validity; however, there is more personal testimony from avid users of ascorbic acid than there is irrefutable evidence. '*C*' also stands for citrus, where this vitamin is found. It could also stand for collagen, the protein 'cement' that is formed with ascorbic acid as a required cofactor. Many foods contain vitamin C, and many important functions are mediated by it as well."[132]

Vitamin C deficiency, the symptoms of which were once considered the result of a contagious disease, has been the arch enemy of armies, navies and explorers throughout history. Known as *scurvy*, vitamin C deficiency was described by ancient peoples, and most notably among those who spent considerable time at sea and away from fresh, vitamin-C bearing foods. Hence, Greeks, Egyptians and Romans made note of the ravages of this seemingly uncontrollable disease from as early as 1500 B.C. Aristotle describes the illness in 450 B.C. "as a syndrome characterized by lack of energy, gum inflammation, tooth decay, and bleeding problems."[133]

---

[132] Haas
[133] ibid.

Essential to collagen formation, vitamin C helps maintain the integrity of substances of mesenchymal (pertaining to the meshwork of embryonic connective tissue in the mesoderm from which are formed the connective tissues of the body, and also the blood vessels and lymphatic vessels) origin, such as connective tissue, osteoid tissue of bone, and dentin of teeth. Vitamin C also participates in the creation of folic acid, absorption of iron and metabolism of amino acids such as *phenylalanine* (essential for optimal growth in infants and for nitrogen equilibrium in human adults) and tyrosine (a precursor of thyroid hormones, catecholamines and melanin).[134]

"In the mid-1500s the Indians of eastern Canada knew that an extract from white cedar needles would cure the disease. An association between citrus fruit and scurvy was first noted in the 16th century when Sir Richard Hawkins observed on his voyage to the South Seas that the sickness could be cured by oranges and lemons. Despite his observation, 10,000 British soldiers died of scurvy that same year. Over 100 years later, James Lind, a Scottish physician serving the British navy, tested various agents for their effectiveness at curing scurvy and reported that two patients given citrus fruits recovered within six days. Despite his study, it was another 48 years before the passage of the Merchant Seaman's Act of 1835 which required that lime or lemon juice be included in the rations of the mercantile service and earned British sailors the name *limeys*."[135]

Elson Haas, M.D. writes, "Ascorbic acid was not isolated from lemons until 1932, though the scourge of scurvy, the vitamin C deficiency disease, has been present for thousands of years. Other cultures of the world discovered their own sources of vitamin C. Powdered rose hips, acerola cherries, or spruce needles were consumed regularly, usually as teas, to prevent the scurvy disease."[136] (Today many vitamin C supplements feature rose hips or acerola on the label, but the consumer is misled into believing that

---

[134] Merck, page 974.
[135] Smolin, pages 300-301.
[136] Haas

these foods are the main sources of vitamin C. In actuality, it is common for isolated vitamin C to be the **main ingredient** with only five or ten percent comprised of rose hips or acerola).

Vitamin C deficiency's resultant scurvy is due to the vitamin's role in the "post translational modification of collagens. Scurvy is characterized by easily bruised skin, muscle fatigue, soft swollen gums, decreased wound healing and hemorrhaging, osteoporosis and anemia." Because vitamin C is readily absorbed, unlike many other nutrients, the symptoms and disease from deficiency are from a lack of the vitamin as opposed to digestive assimilation problems. "The primary physiological state leading to an increased requirement for vitamin C is severe stress (or trauma). This is due to a rapid depletion in the adrenal stores of the vitamin. The reason for the decrease in adrenal vitamin C levels is unclear but may be due either to redistribution of the vitamin to areas that need it or an overall increased utilization."[137]

The best-known sources of vitamin C are citrus fruits—oranges, lemons, limes, tangerines, and grapefruits. Also high in natural concentrations are acerola cherries, rose hips, and, followed by papayas, cantaloupes, and strawberries. However, some ethnobiologists, including James Duke, Ph.D., claim that that there is no greater source of vitamin C than can be found in the rare Amazon rainforest berry known as *camu camu*. This unusual berry-like fruit contains more than twice the amount of vitamin C than found in the highest vitamin C foods of common use in the rest of the so-called "civilized" world. At 2.7 grams of ascorbic acid per 100 grams of fruit, the ascorbic acid content is nothing short of astounding![138] At this writing, however, it is difficult to obtain camu camu for supplementation, as the fruit is considerably difficult to store for transportation and subject

---

[137] King

[138] "Natural food-Fruit Vitamin C Content": The Natural Food Hub, re: Romero, M.A,. Rodriguez, *et al* 'Determination of Vitamin C and Organic acids in various fruits by HPLC', *Journal of Chromatographic Science, Vol 30, Nov 1992, pages 433-437*

to oxidation and mold. This is owing primarily to the intense humidity and heat of the rainforest where it must be harvested.

"Good vegetable sources [of vitamin C] include red and green peppers (the best), broccoli, Brussels sprouts, tomatoes, asparagus, parsley, dark leafy greens, cabbage, and sauerkraut. There is not much available in the whole grains, seeds, and beans; however, when these are sprouted, their vitamin C content shoots up. Sprouts, then, are good foods for winter and early spring, when other fresh fruits and vegetables are not as available. Animal foods contain almost no vitamin C; though fish, if eaten raw, has enough to prevent deficiency symptoms."[139]

Vitamin C, as a weak acid, may become depleted in the presence of alkalis such as baking soda. It is also easily oxidized in the presence of oxygen, and is sensitive to light and heat (including pasteurization). In the diet, vitamin C may be easily lost due to cooking from temperature, exposure to air and in cooking water (as a water-soluble vitamin contained in watery portions of fruits and vegetables). Too much copper in water pipes or cooking pots may also diminish vitamin C content.

Haas writes, "Vitamin C is a very complex and important vitamin." Yet, in defiance of this fact, "ascorbic acid" is a name that has become interchangeable with vitamin C despite that vitamin C, in its food state, is a complex containing **more than just ascorbic acid.**

> "Ascorbic acid is derived from glucose via the uronic acid pathway. The enzyme *l-gulonolactone oxidase* responsible for the conversion of gulonolactone to ascorbic acid is absent in primates, making ascorbic acid required in the diet. The active form of vitamin C is ascorbate acid. The main function of ascorbate is as a reducing agent in a number of different reactions. Vitamin C has the potential to reduce cytochromes A and C of the respiratory chain as well as molecular oxygen. The most important reaction

---

[139] Haas

requiring ascorbate as a cofactor is the hydroxylation [introducing the hydroxyl group to] of proline [an amino acid formed by the decomposition of proteins] residues in collagen. Vitamin C is, therefore, required for the maintenance of normal connective tissue as well as for wound healing since synthesis of connective tissue is the first event in wound tissue remodeling. Vitamin C also is necessary for bone remodeling due to the presence of collagen in the organic matrix of bones."[140]

As a cofactor, vitamin C is involved in other metabolic reactions, including the catabolism of tyrosine and the synthesis of epinephrine from tyrosine, and the synthesis of bile acids. "It is also believed that vitamin C is involved in the process of steroidogenesis since the adrenal cortex contains high levels of vitamin C which are depleted upon adrenocorticotropic hormone (ACTH) stimulation of the gland."[141]

Doubtless, as with other vitamins, ascorbic acid alone has yielded astounding "results" when used as a synthetic substance, showing promise in studies against cancer, the common cold, low immunity, and constipation, to name only a few. However, these results are pharmacological (in using the synthetic vitamin against specific diseases or symptoms), and few studies concentrate on any nutrient depletion that may occur as a result of isolated ascorbic acid's presence and action upon the body's biochemistry. In terms of ascorbic acid yielding a nutrient effect, some researchers boldly argue that this is not even possible because ascorbic acid alone is not a nutrient, but rather a chemical, missing all of the natural cofactors needed to be a complex *bio*chemical.

"Vitamin C…is not stored appreciably in our body, and most excess amounts are eliminated rapidly through the urine. However, amounts over 10 grams per day that some people use and some doctors prescribe are associated with some side effects, though none that are serious. Diarrhea is the

[140] ibid.
[141] ibid.

most common and usually is the first sign that the body's tissue fluids have been saturated with ascorbic acid. Most people will not experience this with under 5–10 grams per day, the amount that is felt to correlate with the body's need and use. Other side effects [may] include nausea, dysuria (burning with urination), and skin sensitivities (sometimes sensitivity to touch or just a mild irritation). Hemolysis (breakage) of red blood cells may also occur with very high amounts of vitamin C. With any of these symptoms, it is wise to decrease intake."[142] Symptomatology is a sign of one or more imbalances, an argument against overdose, superdose and excessive dosaging.

Some ascorbic acid is stored in the body, where it seems to concentrate in the organs of higher metabolic activity. These include the adrenal glands (about 30 mg), pituitary, brain, eyes, ovaries, and testes. Some sources claim that most people require at least 200 mg of vitamin C (as ascorbic acid) a day in the diet to maintain body stores—much more if one smokes, drinks alcohol, or is under stress, has allergies, is elderly, or has diabetes.[143]

Vitamin C plays an important role in glandular health and nerve function. Because vitamin C is so closely related to adrenal health and thyroid support (by stimulating the production of thyroxine, T4), it tends to support the biochemistry in fighting fatigue and regulating metabolism.

Tyrosine, a "nonessential" amino acid, is converted into norepinephrine—a neurotransmitter affecting mood and other emotional/psychological states. Tyrosine requires vitamin C to form other neurotransmitter substances such as dopamine and epinephrine (adrenaline). Vitamin C stimulates adrenal function and the release of norepinephrine and epinephrine, frequently referred to as stress hormones. In this way, prolonged stress and adrenal fatigue often lead to vitamin C deficiency, evidenced by decreased blood levels of vitamin C. Birth control pills may also lead to

---

142 ibid.
143 ibid.

vitamin C deficiency, as they lower tyrosine levels. Researchers speculate that this may be related to cases of depression caused by use of the Pill.[144]

In addition to aiding in the metabolism of tyrosine, vitamin C also works to metabolize folic acid and tryptophan. The latter is converted in the presence of ascorbic acid to 5-hydroxytryptophan to form serotonin, an important brain chemical. Vitamin C helps folic acid convert to its active form, tetrahydrofolic acid. Vitamin C also plays a role in lowering blood cholesterol and acting as an antioxidant.

Working with other vitamins, vitamin C protects vitamins A, B and E from oxidation. Research has shown that ascorbic acid is a detoxifier that may reduce the side effects of several drugs, including cortisone, aspirin and insulin. Further, it may play a role in reducing the toxicity of certain metals such as lead, mercury and arsenic. Vitamin C aids in the body's absorption of iron by helping convert dietary iron to a soluble form. It helps to reduce the ability of food components such as phytates to form insoluble complexes with, and reduce the absorption of, iron. Vitamin C decreases the absorption of copper. Calcium and manganese supplements may decrease vitamin C excretion, and vitamin C supplements may increase manganese absorption. Vitamin C also helps to reduce folic acid excretion. Vitamin C deficiency may lead to increased excretion of vitamin B_6. Vitamin C helps protect against the toxic effects of cadmium, copper, vanadium, cobalt, mercury and selenium.

Many studies have reported the immune-boosting effects of vitamin C, with potential to prevent and ward off infections, flu, respiratory disease and other illnesses. In respiratory disease such as pneumonia, vitamin C is important in supporting the strength/elasticity of lung tissue linings to keep the lungs from collapsing. Research shows that vitamin C also works to activate neutrophils (the most prevalent white blood cells), as well as increase production of lymphocytes (white blood cells important

---

[144] Lininger, page 51, re: Rose, DP, Cramp, DG. Reduction of plasma tyrosine by oral contraceptives and estrogens: a possible consequence of tyrosine amino-transferase induction. *Clin Chem Acta* 1970;29; 49-53.

in antibody production), and coordinating cellular immune function. Further, vitamin C may reduce the production of histamine to fight the effects of irritants commonly called allergens.

The RDA (recommended daily allowance) for adults is 60mg of vitamin C. Despite the widespread megadosing, many researchers tell us that we need only from 10 to 20mg to prevent scurvy, which is an amount easily digestible from only one portion of most fruits and vegetables. For decades, scientists have battled over the efficacy of consuming large amounts of ascorbic acid, and the debate still continues. A recent study reported in the *Journal of Clinical Nutrition* suggested that doses of vitamin C above 200 mg do not increase blood levels of the vitamin significantly and may be excreted. Researchers at the University of Tucson in Arizona measured blood levels of vitamin C when the dose given was 200 mg and then again when 2500 mg was administered. They found negligible increases. As the blood levels of a nutrient typically reflect its effect on the body, the authors of the study feel that megadoses of vitamin C are excreted and have little effect. [145]

Lisa Hark, Ph.D., R.D., reports:

> In a study published in the April 9 issue of *Nature*, Dr. Ian Podman and colleagues from the University of Leicester in England found that vitamin C intake, at levels greater than 500 mg/day may not be advisable. These researchers studied 30 healthy individuals who were given doses of 500 mg/day for a period of 6 weeks. (The RDA for vitamin C is currently 60 mg/day). Results showed oxidative damage at the cellular level even after excess vitamin C was excreted. The authors of this study conclude that high doses of vitamin C may be doing damage to your cells as well. Therefore, it is probably advisable to obtain as much vitamin C from your diet…and limit your vitamin C supplementation to less than 500 mg/day. [146]

---

[145] *Vitamin News*, Dec.1997, re: *The Journal of Clinical Nutrition*
[146] Hark, Ph.D., R.D., Lisa, "Vitamin C: Its Role in Health and Prevention, citing: Podman, Ian, *Nature*, April 9, 1998, (392:559) ; *Eat fruits and vegetables. 5 a Day-for Better Health*. National Cancer Institute. 1998.

Food nutrient researchers are continually trying to agree on an ideal minimum of vitamin C needed on a daily basis. Whereas some researchers refuse to budge beyond the 60mg (RDA) range, others, like Pauling, are to be found in the megadose range—recommending anywhere from 5 to 13 grams daily and more. One standardized test for how much ascorbic acid should be used for supplementation is to take the vitamin in its crystalline/synthetic form in amounts necessary to cause diarrhea and then backing off the amount at the level where such sickness abates.

"Megadoses of vitamin C of 1000-2000 mg have commonly been associated with gastrointestinal disturbances (nausea, abdominal cramps and diarrhea). In general, megadoses of vitamin C should be avoided in individuals with a history of renal stones due to oxalate formation or hemochromatosis or other diseases related to excessive iron accumulation. Excess vitamin C may predispose premature infants to hemolytic anemia due to the fragility of their red blood cells."[147]

Despite the 200mg (University of Tucson study, above) and 60mg (RDA) levels mentioned, a few scientists of late have determined that the *optimum* intake of ascorbic acid is 500mg per day. Recent tests on healthy males indicate 200mg per day is required to maintain tissues at full saturation, but without excreting vitamin C. Another point-of-view hails from researchers studying eating habits, patterns and nutrient intakes of ancient hunter-gatherers. These researchers claim that dietary considerations were once dependent largely upon on the season, the particular ecosystem the tribe was living in, and the size of the family unit that shared whatever resource was available. Researchers Romero and Rodriguez, in their study "Determination of Vitamin C and Organic Acids in Various Fruits" (1992), state: "The daily intake [in early human, prehistoric diets] would probably have been well in excess of the RDA at times of year when fruit

---

[147] American Society for Nutritional Sciences, re: Gershoff, S.N. (1993) Vitamin C (ascorbic acid): new roles, new requirements? *Nutr. Rev.* 51: 313-326 ; Diplock, A.T. (1995) Safety of antioxidant vitamins and b-carotene. *Am. J. Clin. Nutr.* 62: 1510S-1516S.

and greens were relatively abundant, and at other times may well have been much less. Either way, it is unlikely we took in 500 mg per day every day. The 500 mg so-called 'optimum' probably reflects the need for a city living human to protect against stressful living, and the now wide exposure to damaging environmental chemicals. **Such a level can only realistically be obtained by taking supplemental vitamin C...**"[148] Although the word "supplementation" is bandied about in relation to vitamin C and other vitamins, the form of supplementation is not restricted merely to synthetic vitamin C/ascorbic acid. Rather, many nutrition practitioners rely instead on whole food concentrate supplements which supply vitamin C foods in a concentrated form. In this regard, vitamin C is being ingested in its original food complex along with cofactors needed by the body to metabolize and balance vitamin C, as well as other nutrient supplies. "Nutritionists generally regard any 'serving' of food that provides 10 percent to 25 percent of the daily vitamin C need in a relatively low calorie package as a 'good' source. The serving size most of us choose is pretty uniform—most of us would eat one apple, half an avocado in a salad, half a medium sized tomato as part of a salad, one banana, a slice of melon, and so on. On this basis, some fruits, such as kiwi fruit, are quite outstanding, in that they provide more than the RDA in one relatively small fruit."[149]

Elson Haas, M.D. states that, [in general], infants require about 35mg of vitamin C, with pregnant mothers needing about 80mg and lactating mothers requiring 100mg. Vitamin C needs are increased with stress, pregnancy, environmental and food toxicity and with the use of many prescription and over-the-counter drugs, including aspirin, the Pill, estrogen drugs and cortisone. Nicotine and estrogen have the

---

[148] Romero, M.A,. Rodriguez, *et al* 'Determination of Vitamin C and Organic acids in various fruits by HPLC' *Journal of Chromatographic Science, Vol 30, Nov 1992, pages 433-437* : "Natural food-Fruit Vitamin C Content," The Natural Food Hub, 1999.
[149] ibid.

tendency to increase copper blood levels; when copper is in excess, vitamin C deficiency may occur.[150]

Vitamin C in Cardiovascular Health

Vitamin C's role in preventing heart attacks is predicated on the vitamin's ability to strengthen vascular walls, as well as its antioxidant value. Results of a recent study in Finland, reported in the *British Medical Journal*, suggested that vitamin C deficiency may increase heart attack risk more than three-fold. Researchers from the University of Kuopio measured vitamin C status of more than 1,600 middle aged men between the years 1984 and 1992. During this period more than 13 percent of the men lacking in vitamin C suffered heart attacks compared with 3.8 percent of those with adequate vitamin C. It was theorized that the protective effects of vitamin C are owing to its ability to act as an antioxidant and protect against the build up of atherosclerotic plaque. Results of the study also suggested that blood vitamin C levels above the minimum necessary to prevent deficiency did not lead to any risk reduction. The researchers felt that the use of vitamin C supplements would probably not reduce heart attack risk.

Regarding cardiovascular disease, Matthias Rath, M.D. warns: "The wall of a blood vessel is made of collagen. Therefore, when you run out of ascorbate [vitamin C], it is only a matter of time until that wall of collagen breaks down, is not repaired, cracks open and you bleed to death."[151]

Considering the above, then, vitamin C deficiency may be the first step in arterial/cardiovascular disease. Contrary to the modern-day cholesterol phobia, cholesterol is the body's next line of defense in this nutritionally induced physiological breakdown. Rath explains, "When a crack develops in a blood vessel wall due to a shortage of ascorbate, certain fat packages in the blood have the ability to plug the leak by forming a kind of plaster cast. These packages of fat are known as cholesterol, lipids, low density

---

[150] Haas
[151] Rath, M.D., Mattthias; 1999 *The Doctors' Medical Library*

lipoproteins (LDL), and one especially effective leak plugger, lipoprotein(a), a special type of LDL. LDL is a bag of several thousand cholesterol and other fat molecules, with the bag itself made of protein. In itself, despite all the hype in the media, ordinary LDL is no problem. However, there is one type of LDL, namely lipoprotein(a) which has an extra protein cover on the outside of the usual protein cover. Lipoprotein(a) is a double bag of fat. This outer bag is called apoprotein(a) or apo(a). The 'a' could well stand for *adhesive*, because it is a very sticky substance. When a crack develops in the wall of a blood vessel, this sticky double-bagged fat sack finds its way through the crack. Once there, the apo(a) adhesive outer bag glues it down and begins the process of plugging the leak."[152] The good news is that this avoids death by scurvy; but the bad news is that it sets the stage for blood vessel disease.

"Once having plugged the leak the apo(a) outer bag sticks to whatever other bags of cholesterol (i.e. LDL) float by and glues them down as well. The process looks like the following:

1. The scorbutic (ascorbate deficient) crack in the blood vessel wall is the first step in atherosclerosis.
2. The plugging of the leak with lipoprotein(a) is the second step.
3. The gluing down of other LDL (single layer bags of cholesterol and lipids which are not sticky in themselves) is the third step.
4. The fourth step is the stimulation, by lipoprotein(a), of the muscle cells in the artery wall to multiply, thus forming a tumor (swelling).
5. Then the cleanup crew arrives, also known as macrophages, and they try to eat the whole mess and carry it away. However, many of them overeat, get fat, and become part of the problem by dying and being glued down into the plaque. Because they contain so much fat, they appear under the microscope to be full of foam, and they are therefore known as 'foam cells.'"[153]

---

[152] ibid.
[153] ibid.

In conclusion

Few experts would argue that vitamin C is a substance capable of wondrous effects, biochemically speaking. Yet without its cofactors, vitamin C, as the isolated chemical known as ascorbic acid, is actually only a small part of a greater network of synergists required by the body for myriad biochemical activities. An ascorbic acid pill contains none of the synergists and cofactors found in whole foods, and when taken as a supplement, the body is left to manage without these needed, but ignored, nutrients.

VITAMIN D COMPLEX
& SYNERGISTIC COMPOSITION

Like any other vitamin, vitamin D is never found alone in nature, and is a complex that works interdependently as "a member of a large and cooperative bone-making and bone-maintenance **team** made up of nutrients and other compounds."[154] Vitamin D is dependent upon vitamin A, vitamin C, hormones parathormone and calcitonin, collagen and minerals such as calcium, phosphorus, magnesium, and fluoride—composing the inorganic part of bone. Vitamin D is metabolized in the liver and then in the kidney where it is then considered to be the biologically functioning form of vitamin D. The major functions of vitamin D are to increase the efficiency of intestinal calcium absorption and to mobilize calcium stores from bone to maintain the serum calcium and phosphorus concentrations within the normal physiological range.

The richest food sources of vitamin D include fish oils, such as cod or halibut, and the flesh of oily fish such as sardines, salmon and mackerel, as well as some breads and cereal, and some egg yolks. Milk is also a good source of vitamin D when raw. Recent evidence suggests that the vitamin D content in milk is variable and 50 percent of milk samples tested did not contain at least 50 percent of what was stated on the label. Some milk samples do not contain any vitamin D. The results of such surveys may be attributable to the destruction of vitamin D due to pasteurization (which also destroys important enzyme activity in milk and dairy products). Most

---

[154] Whitney, page 253.

milk products therefore, are fortified with isolated vitamin D. Biochemistry teaches that "milk is not a very good source of vitamin D, although its vitamin D content may be increased by irradiation (natural, not to be confused with food irradiation) with ultraviolet light. The vitamin D content of the body may be increased by exposure of the skin to ultraviolet rays from the sun, but care must be taken to avoid overexposure and consequent sunburn. For this reason, vitamin D is sometimes called 'the sunshine vitamin.'"[155]

Vitamin D is well known for its ability to prevent rickets in children and *osteomalacia* in adults. Sunshine seems to be the most important element in rickets prevention because of its unique role in the synthesis of *calciferol* (vitamin D_2) in the skin. Calciferol is classified as a hormone, as it is present in small amounts in the body, and may be present in adequate quantities in natural foods. It is formed in the skin (far removed from target organs), its rate of synthesis (or dietary intake) requires careful control, and its mechanism of action, like that of the estrogens, may be linked to DNA-directed processes. "Another reason for considering calciferol as a hormone is that it is closely linked with two other hormones, calcitonin and the parathyroid hormone, in the control of the calcium level in the blood."[156]

Rickets is characterized by improper mineralization during the development of the bones, resulting in soft bones. Restated, rickets is the result of an inability to deposit calcium phosphate in the bones, causing them to become soft and pliable, leading to deformity—wherein joints enlarge and the ribs become beaded—referred to as *rachitic rosary*. Either injections of small amounts of calciferol or one of its derivatives, or adequate exposure to sunlight, has prevented or cured rickets.

Osteomalacia is characterized by demineralization of previously formed bone leading to increased softness and susceptibility to fracture. A diet low in phosphorus and vitamin D may lead to osteomalacia, a rare condition suggesting that adults need less vitamin D than children do. Osteomalacia

---

[155] ibid.
[156] Sackheim, page 429.

is more likely to occur in women after repeated pregnancies and periods of lactation during which there has been a deficiency of vitamin D. In adulthood, a lack of calcium and vitamin D may cause osteoporosis which, like osteomalacia, is characterized by decalcification and softening of the bones, but to a much greater extent.[157] Vitamin D deficiency may result in muscle weakness, bony deformities, neuromuscular irritability causing muscle spasms of the larynx (laryngospasm) and hands (carpopedal spasm), generalized convulsions and tetany. Working to deposit calcium salts into bone and maintain calcium-phosphorus homeostasis, vitamin D is essential not only in the diet, but also, indirectly, from exposure to sunlight.

The active metabolite of vitamin D is *calcitriol* (1,25-dihydroxyvitamin D), also known biochemically as *1,25-dihydroxycholecalciferol*. Bone repair may not take place when calcitrol is insufficient, as calcitrol controls absorption of calcium in the intestine. Another important food constituent that works interactively with vitamin D is *calcitonin*, a peptide hormone produced by the thyroid, parathyroid and thymus glands that increases calcium deposition in the bone and lowers the quantity in the blood. This process is the opposite of the action of parathyroid hormone.[158]

Vitamin D_1, originally called vitamin D, is actually a mixture of vitamins D_2 (ergocalciferol) and D_3 (cholecalciferol) which are co-constituents of the vitamin D complex stored in body fat. Both are referred to, generically speaking, as vitamin D. Vitamin D precursors produced in yeasts and plants (ergosterol) and animals (7-dehydrocholesterol) are converted to vitamin D by exposure to ultraviolet light. "There is mounting evidence that in the absence of any exposure to sunlight the RDA for vitamin D in adults is between 600 and 800 IU (20 µg/day)."[159]

---

[157] Sackheim, page 431.

[158] Gallagher, Christopher J., "The Role of Vitamin D in the pathogenesis and treatment of osteoporosis." *Journal: J Rheumatol* 1996; (suppl 45)23:15-8.

[159] American Society for Nutritional Sciences, 1999, re: Holick, M.F. (1994) Vitamin D-new horizons for the 21st century. *Am. J. Clin. Nutr.* 60:619-630; DeLuca, H.F. (1988) The vitamin D story: a collaborative effort of basic science and clinical medicine. FASEB J. 2:224-236.

Calcitriol functions in concert with parathyroid hormone (PTH) and calcitonin to regulate serum calcium and phosphorous levels. PTH is released in response to low serum calcium and induces the production of calcitriol. In contrast, reduced levels of PTH stimulate synthesis of inactive vitamin D to its active form. In the intestinal epithelium, calcitriol functions as a steroid hormone in inducing the expression of a protein (calbindinD28K) involved in intestinal calcium absorption. Increased absorption of calcium ions requires concomitant absorption of a negatively charged counter ion to maintain electrical neutrality. The role of calcitonin in balancing levels of calcium is to decrease elevated serum calcium levels by inhibiting bone resorption.[160]

Active calcitriol is derived from ergosterol (produced in plants) and from 7-dehydrocholesterol (produced in the skin). Ergocalciferol (vitamin D2) is formed by ultraviolet irradiation of ergosterol. In the skin, 7-dehydrocholesterol is converted to cholecalciferol (vitamin D3) following ultraviolet irradiation (exposure of the skin to sunlight). Vitamin D2 and D3 are processed to D2-calcitriol and D3-calcitriol, respectively, by the same enzymatic pathways in the body. Cholecalciferol (or egrocalciferol) is absorbed from the intestine and transported to the liver bound to a specific vitamin D-binding protein. Production of calcitriol occurs through the activity of a specific enzyme (D3-1-hydroxylase) present in the tubules of the kidneys and in bone and placenta. A 1997 study out of Tufts University, Boston, showed that vitamin D levels in winter may lead to an increased risk of bone loss in elderly men and women. Results from this study, published in *The American Journal of Clinical Nutrition* showed that "vitamin D levels decrease in winter and parathyroid hormone levels increase. This may accelerate bone loss. The researchers examined *calcidiol* (25-hydroxyvitamin D) concentrations in 182 men and 209 women aged over 65. Levels were found to be lower in women. In wintertime levels were lower than in

---

[160] American Society for Nutritional Sciences 1999; Holick, M.F. (1994) Vitamin D-new horizons for the 21st century. Am. J. Clin. Nutr. 60:619-630 ; DeLuca, H.F. (1988) The vitamin D story: a collaborative effort of basic science and clinical medicine. FASEB J. 2:224-236.

summertime. Travel, vitamin D intake and time spent outdoors increased the calcidiol concentrations.[161]

As with any isolated vitamin, excessive intake may lead to toxic states and symptomatology. Excessive quantities of vitamin D (more than 5,000-10,000 IU/day) have been studied to cause hypercalcemia, hypercalciuria, kidney stones, and soft tissue calcifications.[162]

Vitamin D supplementation alone (as an isolate), although highly touted in its role in bone health, may not provide as much benefit as once predicted. The results of one recent study, reported in *Annals of Internal Medicine*, regarding the relationship between vitamin D intake and bone fractures in elderly people, has found that supplements did not reduce the incidence of fractures. "The study which was carried out in Amsterdam looked at the effects of either vitamin D or a placebo on 2,500 healthy men and women over the age of 70 who were living independently. The participants received a placebo or a daily dose of 400 IU of vitamin D for a three and a half year period. Dietary calcium intake was the same in both groups. 48 fractures were observed in the placebo group and 58 in the vitamin D group. Previous studies have found that vitamin D supplements do reduce the incidence of fractures. The researchers explain that this may be due to the better health of the participants of this study than those of previous studies. It may also be the case that vitamin D supplements may be more effective in older, frailer people."[163]

---

[161] *Vitamin News*, April /May 1997, re: *The Journal of Clinical Nutrition*, 1996
[162] ibid.
[163] *Vitamin Update*, July 1996, re: Annals of Internal Medicine, 124, 400-406.

VITAMIN E COMPLEX
& SYNERGISTIC COMPOSITION

Vitamin E is a complex of fat-soluble substances including eight naturally occurring compounds in two classes designated as tocopherols and tocotrienols. "Each of these compounds exhibits different biological activities. *d*-a-Tocopherol has the highest biological activity and is the most widely available form of vitamin E in food. The other isomers (b, g, d), some of which are more abundant in a typical Western diet, are less biologically active than *d*-a-tocopherol. The commercially available **synthetic** forms of vitamin E are comprised of approximately an equal mixture of eight stereoisomeric forms of a-tocopherol. For practical purposes, 1 international unit (IU) of vitamin E is referred to as 1 mg of the synthetic form, *racemic a-tocopherol acetate*, and the natural form of d-a-tocopherol has a biopotency of vitamin E equal to 1.49 IU."[164]

Michael King, Ph.D., medical biochemist, Indiana State University, explains,

---

[164] American Society for Nutritional Sciences: Meydani, M. (1995) Vitamin E. *Lancet* 345: 170-175 Meydani, S.N., Wu, D., Santos, M.S. & Hayek, M.G. (1995) Antioxidants and immune response in aged persons: Overview of present evidence. Am. J. Clin. Nutr.; 62: 1463S-1462S ; Miller, R.D. & Hayes, K.C. (1982) Vitamin excess and toxicity. In: *Nutritional Toxicology* (Hathcock, J.N., ed.) vol. 1, pp. 81-133. Academic Press, New York, NY.

"The a-tocopherol molecule is the most potent of the tocopherols. Vitamin E is absorbed from the intestines packaged in *chylomicrons*. It is delivered to the tissues via chylomicron transport and
then to the liver through chylomicron remnant uptake. The liver
can export vitamin E in VLDLs [very low density lipoproteins].
Due to its lipophilic [affinity for fat] nature, vitamin E accumulates
in cellular membranes, fat deposits and other circulating lipoproteins. The major site of vitamin E storage is in adipose [fat] tissue.
The major function of vitamin E is to act as a natural **antioxidant** by
scavenging free radicals and molecular oxygen. In particular vitamin
E is important for preventing peroxidation of polyunsaturated
membrane fatty acids. The vitamins E and C are interrelated in their
antioxidant capabilities. Active a-tocopherol can be regenerated by
interaction with vitamin C following scavenge of a peroxy free radical. Alternatively, a-tocopherol can scavenge two peroxy free radicals
and then be conjugated to glucuronate for excretion in the bile."[165]

Vitamin E as a supplement is at best incomplete, and like all other isolated substances, at worst it is a synthetic chemical compound. About 75
percent of the vitamin E found in food is the *gamma tocopherol* form, while
supplements may not contain any gamma tocopherol. Taking very high
doses of alpha tocopherol may displace gamma tocopherol.[166]

Vitamin E's most sought-after effect is as an antioxidant and is
regarded as "the most effective chain-breaking lipid-soluble antioxidant
in the biological membrane, where it contributes to membrane stability.
It protects critical cellular structures against damage from oxygen free
radicals and reactive products of lipid peroxidation."[167]

---

[165] Michael W. King, Ph.D, Terre Haute Center for Medical Education,
Indiana State University Department of Biochemistry, November 1999.
[166] *Vitamin News* for April/May 1997
[167] ibid

Vitamin E deficiency is most noted in reproductive failure, nutritional "muscular dystrophy," hemolytic anemia, and neurological and immunological abnormalities. Vitamin E is known to prevent sterility in animals; and some animals on a vitamin E-deficient diet have developed muscular dystrophy resulting in paralysis.[168]

Vitamin E deficiency may lead to shortened length of RBC [red blood cell] life. "Edema and flaky dermatitis have been associated with low plasma E, as has increased peroxide hemolysis in premature infants on formulas containing vegetable oil. The deficiency state may be diagnosed when the plasma tocopherol level is low. RBC susceptibility to hydrogen peroxide is increased with levels <0.5mg/dL[169]

Newer studies have pointed to vitamin E's benefit to cardiac and skin tissues, although traditional medical literature claims that a vitamin E deficiency occurs rarely in humans, save in cases of premature infants with very low birth weight and patients who fail to absorb fat. With its combined antioxidant potential, including the ability to preserve vitamin A, and benefit to the heart and skin, vitamin E is considered an anti-aging nutrient.

Recent studies show that vitamin E influences signal transduction pathways which may have nothing to do with the antioxidant properties of the vitamin. In vitro studies show that vitamin E influences expression of adhesion molecules on endothelial cells and monocyte adhesion to endothelial cells. High serum vitamin E levels have been associated with reduced risk for coronary heart disease in men and women.[170]

Low vitamin E levels may be linked with angina related to coronary artery spasm. Japanese researchers at Toyama University measured plasma vitamin E levels and total lipid levels in patients with various types of angina. The conclusion was that patients with active variant angina had

[168] Sackheim, page 432.
[169] Berkow, M.D., Robert, Editor, *The Merck Manual,* 16th Ed.,, NJ, 1992, page 966.
[170] ibid

vitamin E levels significantly lower than those seen in people with no evidence of coronary artery disease. "The researchers also found that vitamin E levels rose as patients remained free of angina attacks for six months or longer. Variant angina caused by coronary artery spasm can occur when a person is at rest, can happen at odd times of the day or night and is more common in women under the age of 50."[171]

Harvard Medical and Brigham and Women's Hospital in Boston have proclaimed that women supplementing with vitamin E for two years or more reduced their risk of cardiovascular disease by up to 40 percent; similar results were reported for men.[172]

Due to the synergists present in vitamin E-containing foods, some researchers argue that whole food sources are effective where isolated vitamin E supplementation fails. Reported in *HealthNews*:

> Vitamin E's role in heart disease prevention continues to be a hot topic of debate. Last month, we told you about a British study that found a reduced risk of nonfatal heart attack in people who took large doses of vitamin E pills. Now a study in the May 2 *New England Journal of Medicine* finds that postmenopausal women who received the most **vitamin E from foods**—about 10 IU a day—were about 60 percent less likely to die of heart disease than those whose intake of the vitamin was lowest (about 5 IU). **Supplements appeared to have no effect.** Even without a definitive answer, it still makes sense to get at least the RDA (30 IU) of

[171] *Circulation* 1996, 94.

[172] Garrison, MA, R.Ph., Robert and Elizabeth Somer, MA, RD, *The Nutrition Desk Reference,* Keats Publishing, CT, 1995; reporting: Rimm E., Ascherio A, Willet W, et. all: Vitamin E supplementation and risk of coronary heart disease among men (Meeting Abstract), *Circulation,* 1992; 86:463.; Stampfer M, Hennekens C, Manson J, et. all: Vitamin E consumption and the risk of coronary disease in women. *New England Journal of Medicine,* 1993; 328: 1444-1449.

vitamin E from food. Good sources include seeds and nuts, vegetable oils, wheat germ, tuna fish, and oatmeal. [173]

As an antioxidant, vitamin E competes with air pollution to affect the health of skin tissue:

"Recent findings from a study reported at the annual meeting of the Oxygen Club of California suggest that the ozone found in air pollution may remove vitamin E from the uppermost layer of the skin. This can lead to an aggravation of skin problems such as eczema and psoriasis. Researchers at the University of California exposed the skin for two hours to ozone levels twice those of peak times for heavily smog-polluted regions. They then measured the vitamin E content of the skin and found that a reduction of up to 25 percent. After a similar exposure for six consecutive days only about one quarter of the original vitamin E remained. Previous scientific studies have shown that skin problems worsen in highly polluted areas. The effect on vitamin E may offer an explanation. Vitamin E acts as an antioxidant and protects against free radical damage. Loss of vitamin E may lead to the breakdown of fat molecules which regulate the movement of substances in and out of the skin. This breakdown may also trigger inflammatory responses in the lower layers of the skin." [174]

As time goes by, studies continue to elucidate vitamin E's role in biochemistry, showing that this vitamin complex provides a multitude of health benefits affecting behavior, menopausal symptoms, hormonal balance, skin health, cardiovascular function, cellular protection, intellect and brain function.

---

[173] Vitamin E from Foods May Reduce Women's Heart Disease Risk, *HealthNews* from the publishers of the *New England Journal of Medicine,* June 4, 1996; OnHealth, 2000 OnHealth Network Company
[174] *Vitamin News* for April/May 1997

Austrian researchers assessed vitamin E levels and intellectual function in nearly 1800 adults aged from 50 to 75 to discover that the vitamin may prevent age-related decline in brain function. Reported in the *Journal of the American Geriatrics Society*, 1998, the study showed that those with higher vitamin E levels were less likely to have low scores on tests of intellectual capacity. Such tests are used to assess decline in Alzheimer's disease and other types of dementia.[175]

Vitamin E Food Factors & Selenium

There are many studies performed on the efficacy of isolated vitamin E supplementation against disease, but scant research exists on vitamin E-containing foods wherein the vitamin E complex coexists with its natural cofactors. However, although few in number, the latter studies indicate that vitamin E-containing foods lower the risk of disease. At this writing, researchers can only speculate that it is the entire combination of vitamins, minerals and other dietary (as opposed to supplemental) nutrients that take credit for any salubrious results. For instance, a long-term Nurses Health Study beginning in 1976 proclaimed that eating nuts reduces heart disease risk. This study suggests that women who frequently include nuts in their diet have a reduced risk of coronary heart disease. Involving more than 80,000 women aged from 34 to 59 who had not been diagnosed with any kind of heart disease, researchers collected detailed information on the medical histories and lifestyles of nurses. Every two years, the women receive a follow-up questionnaire. During the 14-year follow-up period for this part of the study, there were 861 cases of non-fatal heart attack and 394 cases of fatal coronary heart disease. Analysis of the results showed that women who ate more than five ounces (approximately 150g) of nuts per week had a 35 percent lower risk of coronary heart disease than women who ate no nuts ate less than 1 ounce (approximately 30g) per month.

---

[175] *Journal of the American Geriatrics Society* 1998;46:1407-10: from *Vitamin News* March 1999.

Results from the Physicians Health Study, reported at the annual meeting of the American Heart Association, also suggest that nuts can reduce the risk of death from heart attack. The results of this study, which lasted for 11 years and involved more than 22,000 male doctors, show that "the risk of total and sudden heart attack decreased with increasing nut consumption."[176] Nuts contain a wide array of nutrients and are known to have beneficial effects on blood fats, decreasing total cholesterol and LDL cholesterol levels. The study proclaimed that the benefits of eating nuts was owing to their potentially protective compounds which include not only vitamin E, but also magnesium, selenium, protein, fiber, potassium and alpha linolenic acid. The results of this study support the efficacy of vitamin E as nutrient component of whole food with its complement of synergistic nutrients intact.

As with many other nutrients, vitamin E deficiency may occur secondarily, by way of digestive difficulties, i.e., malabsorption syndrome, as in cases of sprue, celiac disease, cystic fibrosis or biliary atresia (congenital absence or closure of a normal body orifice or tubular organ).[177]

Food sources of vitamin E, in its entire, naturally occurring complex, include wheat germ and wheat germ oil, as well as in the oils of most grains and seeds (including sunflower). Other sources include milk, eggs, fish, muscle meats, cereals, leafy vegetables and oils such as cottonseed, corn, palm and peanut. J.E. Meyers Botanical Gardens of Hammond, Indiana, reports that watercress is one of the best sources of vitamin E. Dried watercress may contain triple the amount of vitamin E found in dried lettuce leaves.[178] The value of vitamin E in any food, however, must be considered in the raw state, as this vitamin is subject to oxidation and destruction in the presence of ultraviolet light, refining, extreme heating and processing.

---

[176] *British Medical Journal* 1998;317:1341-45 ; from *Vitamin News* March 1999.

[177] Merck, page 966.

[178] Hutchens, Alma R., *Indian Herbology of North America*, Shambhala, Boston, 1991, page 293.

One of the most important cofactors in vitamin E foods is selenium, a celebrated antioxidant mineral. Herbalist James Duke, Ph.D. states that the average Brazil nut (a vitamin E food) contains the Daily Value for selenium (70mg).[179]

The importance of vitamin E in foods is understated in light of today's processed diet and exposure to environmental toxins. The many antioxidant, cancer and cardiovascular studies underway show great interest in the protective value of not only of vitamin E, but also of the foods wherein this vitamin is contained (because of the existing synergists). As part of the vitamin E complex, essential fatty acids (as well as selenium) are important cofactors not to be overlooked. "The major symptom of vitamin E deficiency in humans is an increase in red blood cell fragility. Since vitamin E is absorbed from the intestines in chylomicrons [mainly triglyceride fat particles], any fat malabsorption diseases can lead to deficiencies in vitamin E intake. Neurological disorders have been associated with vitamin E deficiencies associated with fat malabsorptive disorders. Increased intake of vitamin E is recommended in premature infants fed formulas that are low in the vitamin as well as in persons consuming a diet high in polyunsaturated fatty acids. Polyunsaturated fatty acids tend to form free radicals upon exposure to oxygen and this may lead to an increased risk of certain cancers."[180]

Regarding the vitamin E co-nutrient selenium, the American Society for Nutritional Sciences reports:

> Selenium (Se) is an essential trace element that functions as a component of enzymes involved in antioxidant protection and thyroid hormone metabolism...Selenium deprivation reduces activities of the selenium-dependent peroxidases and deiodinases. The signs in animals depend upon vitamin E status and appear

---

[179] Duke, *The Green Pharmacy*, page 24.
[180] King

only when both nutrients are limiting. They vary according to species. For example, selenium-and vitamin E-deficient animals show myopathies of skeletal (e.g., sheep, cow, horse), cardiac (pig) or smooth (dog, cow) muscle; hepatic necrosis (rat, pig); increased capillary permeability (chicken); or pancreatic acinar degeneration (chicken). Characteristic signs of selenium deficiency have not been described in humans, but very low selenium status is a factor in the etiologies of a juvenile cardiomyopathy (Keshan Disease) and a chondrodystrophy (Kaschin-Beck Disease) that occur in selenium-deficient regions of China.[181]

Important sources of selenium are mostly in "vitamin E foods": meats, fish and grains. As stated, of particular note are Brazil nuts, known to have relatively high selenium concentrations. Recent research on selenium points to its anti-tumorigenic effects, yet, "The mechanism(s) of anti-tumorigenic effects of selenium and the possible role of selenium in affecting the risk of human cancer are not clear."[182]

---

[181] American Society for Nutritional Sciences, 1999, re: Burk, R.F., ed. (1994) Selenium in Biology and Human Health. Springer-Verlag, New York, NY; Combs, G.F., Jr. (1994) Essentiality and toxicity of selenium: a critique of the Recommended Dietary Allowances and the Reference Dose. In: Risk Assessment of Essential Elements (Mertz, C., Abernathy, C. & Olin, S.S., eds.), pp. 167-183. International Life Sciences Institute Press, Washington, DC.

[182] ibid

Vitamin F:
Essential Fatty Acids

Volumes have been published on the value and nutrient effects of essential fatty acids, but for the sake of this discussion on whole food complexes, we'll merely offer a glimpse into this most-celebrated food factor that is sometimes referred to as vitamin F.

Essential fatty acids, as implied by the name, are essential to human health, biochemistry, cellular health and physiology. They are involved in energy production, transmission of nerve impulses, cell membrane composition and formation, brain and thinking functions, transfer of oxygen from the air to the bloodstream, the manufacture of hemoglobin, skin health and hormonal function. We cannot survive without ingestion and utilization of raw, natural and whole food fats.

Fats are found in both animal (such as butter, meat, fish and cheese) and plant foods (vegetable oils such as coconut, olive, flax, wheat germ, sunflower, sesame). However, in the modern diet, real, raw and healthy fats from foods have given way to altered fats—fats changed in their molecular structure to unhealthy fats and oils via food processing, hydrogenation, cooking, barbecuing, synthesization and rancidity via oxidation (exposure to air, oxygen). Cooked foods are the mainstay of the modern diet, making adequate amounts of fats, in their original healthy form, a rarity. Even wholesome fats in raw milk and butter have all but disappeared from the diet as political influences have illegalized raw dairy products under the pretense that they are dangerous due to bacterial contamination. This is a weak argument in light of the fact that raw dairy has been the staple and sustenance of human life for thousands of years.

Symptoms of essential fatty acid deficiency may include fatigue, dry skin, immune deficiency, chronic fatigue, chronic illness, hypochondria, liver disease, nervous system disorders, attention deficit, growth retardation, sterility and hormonal dysfunction, mental disease, gastrointestinal disorders and heart and circulatory abnormalities. Fat soluble vitamins are dependent on fats for absorption and metabolism. In foods, essential fatty acids are found right along with their important vitamin cofactors—vitamin E is found in wheat germ oil, vitamin A is found in fish liver oil, vitamin D is found in dairy, etc.

Anthony's Textbook of Anatomy and Physiology states, "An essential fatty acid is one that the body cannot synthesize and that is essential for survival. One's diet, therefore, must include essential fatty acids."[183] There are three essential fatty acids: *arachindonic acid, linoleic acid* (omega-6; polyunsaturated) and *linolenic acid* (omega-3, polyunsaturated). Monosaturated fatty acids are referred to as omega-9s. Saturated fatty acids have their carbon atoms bound to as many hydrogens as possible and therefore contain no carbon-carbon double bonds in their structures. Unsaturated fatty acids contain one or more carbon-carbon double bonds. A monounsaturated fatty acid contains one double bond. A polyunsaturated fatty acid contains more than one double bond.[184]

Fatty acids are named for the location of their double bonds. If the first double bond starts at the third carbon, counting from the CH_3, or methyl end of the chain, the fat is said to be an omega-3 (w-3) fatty acid...If the first double bond starts from the sixth carbon from the CH_3 end, the fatty acid is called an omega-6 (w-6) fatty acid. Most unsaturated fatty acids

[183] Thibodeau, Gary A., *Anthony's Textbook of Anatomy and Physiology* 13th Edition, Times Mirror/Mosby College Publishing, St. Louis, MO, p.42
[184] Smolin, page 134.

found in nature are in the *cis* configuration, having both hydrogen atoms on the same side of the double bond. When the hydrogens are on opposite sides of the double bond, it is a *trans* fatty acid.[185]

Only linoleic acid is actually essential, because the other two fatty acids can be made by the body **if other essential nutrients are provided**. Linoleic acid is found mainly in vegetable oils. Saturated and unsaturated fatty acids differ mainly in how fluid they are. The more saturated a fatty acid is, the more solid it is. Polyunsaturated fatty acids are rich in liquid vegetable oils. An unsaturated fatty acid is one that is generally found in vegetables. Saturated fatty acids are found mainly in animal products.[186]

John Finnegan, author of *The Facts About Fats*, writes:

> Studies have found that the main nutrient most of us are deficient in is the Omega-3 fatty acid. An inadequate intake of this nutrient has been established as a main cause of most modern diseases. Today, because of food processing, the average diet contains only one-sixth the amount needed and one-sixth the amount the average diet contained in 1820. (And in many diets, one-twentieth to one-hundredth the amount needed.)…There are only two main sources of Omega-3 fats: cold water fish oils and organic flaxseed oil. Flaxseed oil is the richer source of Omega-3 fats: it requires less processing, tastes better, contains no toxic substances…, is more stable and is less expensive.

Omega-6 fatty acids are also of critical importance in maintaining good health, although most modern diets contain ample (if not excessive) amounts of Omega-6 fatty acids, but insufficient amounts of Omega-3s. Omega-6s must be taken with an adequate amount of Omega-3s or they can have a deleterious effect on health. An acceptable ratio amount researchers [have determined] is about four to six parts

---

[185] ibid, page 135.
[186] Mosby's Medical Encyclopedia, page 313.

Omega-6 to one part Omega-3 in the diet, yet more primitive diets often point to a one-to-one ratio.

Omega-9 fatty acids are found in olive, hazelnut, sesame and almond oils and have been recognized to benefit liver and gallbladder functions as well as provide energy and prevent heart disease.

Finnegan writes, "Of all the foods that we consume, none is as severely processed and converted into poisonous substances as are the fats and oils. Use of high temperatures and chemical solvents, as well as exposure to light and oxygen in the processing methods of nearly all oils produced today, destroys much of the Omega-3 and-6 essential fatty acids, and creates rancidity, poisonous trans-fatty acids and many other toxic compounds."[187]

Essential Fatty Acids & Prostaglandins

Michael T. Murray, N.D., explains a wide array of effects of essential fatty acids on human biochemistry:

In addition to providing the body with energy, the essential fatty acids—linoleic and linolenic acid—function in our bodies as components of nerve cells, cellular membranes, and **hormone-like substances** known as *prostaglandins*. Prostaglandins and the essential fatty acids play an important role in keeping the body in good working order, such as

- producing steroids and synthesizing hormones
- regulating pressure in the eye, joints or blood vessels
- regulating response to pain, inflammation, and swelling
- mediating immune response
- regulating bodily secretions and their viscosity
- dilating or constricting blood vessels
- regulating collateral circulation

---

[187] Finnegan, John, *The Facts About Fats*, Celestial Arts, Berkeley, CA 1993.

- directing endocrine hormones to their target cells
- regulating smooth muscle and autonomic reflexes
- being primary constituents of cellular membranes
- regulating the rate at which cells divide (mitosis)
- maintaining the fluidity and rigidity of cellular membranes
- regulating in-flow and out-flux of substances in and out of cells
- transporting oxygen from red blood cells to the tissues
- maintaining proper kidney function and fluid balance
- keeping saturated fats mobile in the blood stream
- preventing blood cells from clumping together
- mediating the release of pro-inflammatory substances from cells
- regulating nerve transmission
- stimulating steroid production
- being the primary energy source for the heart muscle[188]

"Other omega-3 fatty acids are manufactured in the body using alpha linolenic acid as a starting point. These include eicosapentaenoic acid (EPA) and docosahexaenoic acid (DHA). Other omega-6 fatty acids can be manufactured in the body using linoleic acid as a starting point. These include gamma-linoleic acid (GLA), dihomogamma-linoleic acid (DHGLA) and arachidonic acid."[189]

Altered Fats, Butter & Disease with the Modern Diet

The role of fats in the diet, in recent times, has been diminished, assaulted and defamed. Political and corporate influences have undermined the importance of fats in the diet to make way for the sale and marketing of

[188] Murray, ND, Michael T., and Jade Beutler, RRT, RCP, *Understanding Fats & Oils*, Progressive Publishing, Encinitas, CA, 1996, pages 1-3.

[189] Reavley, Nicola, *The New Encyclopedia of Vitamins, Minerals, Supplements & Herbs* M. Evans & Company, New York, 1999, pages 330-333.

fake and altered fats which include margarine, Olestra and a host of hydrogenated and partially hyrodgenated oils, "spreads," spray-on oils, etc. The production of altered fats is big business—so big that at one point in the past 30 years one of the most nutritious of all foods—raw butter—has all but disappeared from the dinner table across America.

Blaming real fats for heart disease and death by cholesterol, the altered fats corporations swayed public opinion so far against real fats that to this day the contrived "benefits" of margarine are heralded in schools from elementary level to college and is a mainstay of dietetic teaching. Accusations against butter were not based upon historical usage or medical or scientific fact, but rather political propaganda. To sell their altered fats, manufacturers jumped on the anti-fat bandwagon with the diet craze that also persists to this day by successfully referring to healthy saturated fats as bad fats. In so doing, cholesterol studies have been misinterpreted and the natural foods industry has been slandered.

Much of the bad press on fats centers around cardiovascular illness—one of the most deadly diseases of modern times. Heart disease is frequently blamed on fat consumption, which, though misleading, is great for sales of artificial fats and margarine. "Heart disease was rare in America at the turn of the century. Between 1920 and 1960, the incidence of heart disease rose precipitously to become America's number one killer. During the same period butter consumption plummeted from 18 pounds per person per year to four."[190] As a food, raw butter continues to be an excellent source of vitamin A, E and cholesterol. "A Medical Research Council survey showed that men eating butter ran half the risk of developing heart disease than those using margarine."[191]

---

[190] Fallon, MA, Sally and Mary Enig, Ph.D., "Why Butter is Better," The Price-Pottenger Nutrition Foundation, 1999, Reprinted from *Health Freedom News*, November/December, 1995.

[191] ibid, citing: *Nutrition Week*, March 22, 1991; 21:12:2-3.

These days, a confused public by and large equates fats with health degeneration, obesity, heart disease, high cholesterol, arteriosclerosis and liver complications. Meanwhile, the incidences of cardiovascular disease have risen alongside the sales and proliferation of the altered fats industry. However, fats, like people, can be labeled neither good nor bad without some investigation, prudence and differentiation.

At a 1996, Washington, D.C. news conference, the nonprofit consumer-advocacy group Center for Science in the Public Interest (CSPI) released the results of a major study on the *trans* fat content of brand-name and restaurant foods. The results show that many foods made with partially hydrogenated oil, vegetable shortening, or margarine contain damaging amounts of trans fats. "Trans fat is a secret killer," said Dr. Walter Willett, chairman of the nutrition department at the Harvard School of Public Health. "[Food] labels tell you how much saturated fat you're eating. With trans, it's anybody's guess."[192] Willett's research helped establish the link between trans fat consumption and the risk of heart disease.

Coming down hard on bad fats in the food and restaurant industry, the results of a 41-supermarket and restaurant food study in seven cities across the country published in the September 1996 issue of CSPI's *Nutrition Action Healthletter* reported:

> *French Fries. The hidden trans fat in McDonald's, Hardees, and Arby's fries doubles the damage caused by their saturated fat. Eating a large order of fries at one of those chains is like eating a Quarter Pounder. "They might as well be frying in lard," said [Dr. Mary] Wootan [CSPI researcher]. The fries at Burger King and Wendy's are even worse, she added. "To your arteries, a large order of their fries looks like one and a half Quarter Pounders."

---

[192] Wootan, Dr. Margo, "Trans Fat Spells Double Trouble for Arteries, *What the Food Labels Don't Tell You*," Nutrition Action Healthletter, Center for Science in the Public Interest, 1996.

*Fried Fish. If the trans and saturated fats are added together, Red Lobster's Admiral's Feast dinner contains a two-day supply of artery-clogging fat. "That makes it a coronary from the sea," said Wootan. The dinner includes fried fish, french fries, cole slaw, and garlic bread.

*Fried Chicken. A KFC Original Recipe Dinner (a thigh, drumstick, mashed potatoes, gravy, cole slaw, and a biscuit) has a full day's worth of heart-damaging fat.

*Baked Goods. The trans fat in a plain Dunkin' Donuts Old Fashioned Cake Donut more than doubles the damage its saturated fat inflicts on your heart. Eating just one is like eating eight strips of bacon. Trans fat also increases the amount of harmful fat in many Danish, pies, biscuits, cookies, and crackers.

*Margarine. If full-fat stick margarines like Parkay and Promise had to be honest about their trans fat content, they wouldn't be allowed to claim that they have "70 percent less saturated fat than butter." Claiming "40 percent less" would be more truthful. While that still makes them better for your heart..., the healthiest margarines [an oxymoron] are the ones with the least trans. That means a tub rather than a stick, and a lower-fat margarine.[193]

In the early 1990s, CSPI petitioned the FDA to count trans fat as saturated fat on food labels and asked that the FDA ban claims like "no cholesterol" or "low saturated fat" on foods that are not also low in trans. Dr. Willett, Dr. William Castelli, director of the Framingham Cardiovascular Wellness Institute,Dr. Henry Blackburn, a professor at the University of Minnesota School of Public Health, and other prominent researchers also have urged the FDA to require trans fat labeling. CSPI researchers have since complained that "the FDA has failed to act."[194]

---

[193] ibid
[194] ibid.

Authors Sally Fallon and Mary Enig, Ph.D. explain the role of fats in human health and physiology in relation to their nutritional value in whole, unaltered foods:

> [Healthy] fatty acids are essential parts of all body tissues where they are the major part of the phospholipid component of the cell membrane...When the body does not get enough fat from the diet, it makes fats "from scratch" from carbohydrates. The fatty acids that the body synthesizes are saturated fatty acids—exactly the same kind of saturated fatty acids found in butter, cream and animal fat and monounsaturated fatty acids—exactly the same kind of fatty acids found in olive oil. The cell membranes are composed of a combination of saturated fatty acids, monounsaturated fatty acids and polyunsaturated fatty acids.
>
> It happens that the more fat you consume in your diet, the less your body tissues make from scratch. But when you consume high levels of unnatural polyunsaturated fatty acids such as the kind found in commercial vegetable oils, the normal body synthesis of saturated fat is eliminated and the ingested polyunsaturated fats are used for structural fatty acids, leading to an unnatural balance in the cell membranes.
>
> Essentially it amounts to the following. Low fat, high carbohydrate diets cause the body to make the saturated fatty acids and monounsaturated fatty acids it needs. When the fat that is eaten is mixed and mostly saturated and monounsaturated, it is like the fat the body synthesizes. Under these circumstances, there is no problem with the fatty acid supply that the tissues have available for incorporation into the phospholipids that are an important part of the membrane structure of all cells. On the other hand, when the fat that is eaten is more highly unsaturated, the fatty acids available for incorporation into the tissue phospholipids are more unsaturated than the body normally prefers and this causes

a number of differences in membrane properties that are thought to be detrimental to the regular body economy. High levels of polyunsaturates in the diet have been shown to increase cholesterol levels in tissues, increase fat cell synthesis in growing animals, alter the response of the immune system, increase peroxidation products such as ceroid pigment, increase gallstone formation, and of all things decrease HDL cholesterol in the blood.

Saturated fatty acids have recently been shown to be necessary for the proper utilization of essential fatty acids and for efficient modeling of the bones. Consumption of saturated fatty acids also results in lowering of Lp(a) in the blood. Elevated levels of Lp(a) are a marker for heart disease. The textbooks tell us that saturated fats protect the liver.[195]

In defense of good fats, the *Archives of General Psychiatry* reported in 1999, "Dietary intake of alpha-linolenic acid protects against fatal ischemic heart disease.[196]

The *Journal of Clinical Nutrition,* 1999 reported:

"Results from the Nurses Health Study suggest that dietary intake of the essential fatty acid alpha-linolenic acid is linked to reduced risk of fatal heart disease. The intake of alpha-linolenic acid was determined from a food frequency questionnaire completed in 1984 by over 76,000 women. During 10 years of followup there were 232 cases of fatal ischemic heart disease and 597 non-fatal heart attacks. Analysis of the results showed that a higher intake of alpha-linolenic acid protects against fatal ischemic heart disease. An important source of alpha-linolenic acid is oil and vinegar salad dressing; and women who ate this 5 to 6 times per week

[195] Fallon, MA, Sally and Mary Enig, PhD, The Price-Pottenger Nutrition Foundation, 1999.
[196] *Archives of General Psychiatry,* 1999, ;56: 407-412.

had around half the risk of fatal ischemic heart disease compared to those who rarely did."[197]

The lack of essential fats in the diet leads to a host of malfunctions causing or contributing to a long list of ailments, including (but not limited to) psoriasis, dermatitis, acne, PMS, eczema, sinus conditions, headaches, behavioral disorders, multiple sclerosis, arthritis, heart disease, liver disease, gallbladder disease, hypertension, impotence, vascular (blood vessel) disease, diabetic complications, arteriosclerosis, vision problems and neurological disorders.

Dr. Michael Murray writes:

> Early in the twentieth century, Americans consumed about 125 grams of fat a day. Today, the consumption is closer to 175 grams, a 40 percent increase, or about 50 extra pounds a year. Proportionally our ingestion of saturated fats has remained relatively stable. Our ingestion of unrefined polyunsaturated oils rich in the disease-preventing essential fatty acids has decreased dramatically. Conversely, our ingestion of refined, adulterated polyunsaturated oil products has risen sharply, correlating with the dramatic rise in many degenerative conditions including cancer, heart disease and stroke. These refined and processed compounds actually inhibit the body's ability to use the essential fatty acids that are consumed.[198]

Regarding the introduction of bad fats into the modern diet, nutrition researcher/author Rudolph Ballentine, M.D. writes: by "bubbling hydrogen through vegetable oil," a "new fat" is created…"[A] recent elaborate statistical analysis of the incidence of heart disease and the consumption of hydrogenated fats in England has shown a dramatic and detailed correlation between the two…It is interesting to note that in the Southeastern [United] states, the region where margarine consumption is highest in relation to population and to butter consumption, there is an area where the incidence of

---

[197] *American Journal of Clinical Nutrition* 1999;69:890-897.
[198] Murray.

heart attacks is so high that it has been termed 'an enigma.' It seems increasingly likely that eating margarine, instead of preventing heart attacks, actually accelerates the process which causes them."[199]

Scientists have discovered that when hydrogen is added to vegetable oils, they become solid at room temperature and do not spoil as quickly. This fact is good for business, but bad for human health, as hydrogenated (or partially hydrogenated) oils imbalance the biochemistry, failing to meet the requirements of cells and interfering with natural biochemical processes. Author John Finnegan explains, in the process of hydrogenating oils "natural oils are heated under pressure for six to eight hours at 248-410 degrees F and reacted with hydrogen gas, using a metal-like nickel or copper as a catalyst. If this process is brought to completion, as in vegetable shortening, you have a partially hardened oil, as in most margarines."[200] Trans fatty acids (fatty acids that have been altered molecularly via hydrogenation), writes Finnegan,

> compete for enzymes, produce biologically nonfunctional derivatives and interfere with the work of the essential fatty acids in the body. Because of our association of the word 'polyunsaturates' with health, we are fooled into thinking that we are buying a health-giving product of good quality, a product that is actually health-destroying…There are so many possibilities of different compounds that can be made during partial hydrogenation that they stagger the imagination. Scientists have barely scratched the surface in studying all the changes induced in fats and oils by hydrogenation. Needless to say, the industry is hesitant to fund thorough and systematic studies on the kinds of chemicals produced and their effects on health. The industry is equally hesitant to publicize the information which already exists on the topic.[201]

[199] Ballantine, M.D., Rudolph, *Diet & Nutrition, A Holistic Approach,* 1978. Himalyan International Institute, Homesdale, PA.
[200] Finnegan.
[201] ibid.

The Cholesterol Scare

Beatrice Hunter, Food Editor of Consumers' Research, writes:

> Unquestionably, among all of the food component/health relationships, the fat/cholesterol issue has been the foremost in generating misinformation, confusion, and hoopla. Conclusions of scientific studies have been couched in qualifying phrases such as 'no conclusive evidence,' 'no definite cause-and-effect relationship,' 'uncertainties exist,' 'this finding has yet to be confirmed,' etc. Despite these phrases, tentative findings have become distorted and made to appear as firm facts, and recommendations have been made for dietary and lifestyle changes before a firm scientific base has been established.
>
> The conventional slogans are that fat and cholesterol are bad [and] the less fat and cholesterol one eats, the better for one's health. By cutting down on fat and cholesterol, one lowers the risks of heart disease and cancer...The public has been badly misinformed about the role of fats. Many articles and much advertising characterize all fats as bad...what is ignored is that some fats are essential for health and provide nutrients and palatability to foods...[S]aturated fat and cholesterol in the diet are not the cause of coronary heart disease. That myth is the great- est scientific deception of this century, perhaps of any century. [202]

In 1948, Framingham, Massachusetts, a study was instituted with nearly 30,000 adults to determine the relationships between fats, cholesterol and heart disease. After monitoring their subjects for a number of years, in 1970, the Framingham researchers reported: "There is, in short, no suggestion of any relation between [dietary fat intake] and the subsequent development of

---

[202] Hunter, Beatrice Trum, "Food Health Claims: Fact vs. Fiction," *Consumers' Research*, Washington, DC, May 1991, pp. 10-14.

CHD (coronary heart disease) in the study group."[203] Despite this admission, a vast program was already being developed urging the public to lower cholesterol levels, with "helpful drugs" waiting in the wings for those who could not achieve the required levels. Hunter writes, "By the early 1980s, both the National Heart, Lung and Blood Institute and the American Heart Association concluded that, despite the lack of definite proof, there was sufficient suggestive evidence linking [dietary fat intake] with CHD to launch a nationwide campaign to change American eating habits."[204]

Regardless of the motivation for doing so, taking a stand against cholesterol and fats amounts to ignorance, slander and defiance of biochemical fact, resulting in disease and death beginning at the cellular level.

[203] ibid.
[204] ibid.

Vitamin K:
The Antihemorrhaging Agent

Vitamin K (derived from the first initial of the Danish word *koagulation*, or, in English, coagulation) is a nutrient complex comprised of three components: vitamin K_1 (philloquinone, phylloquinone or hytonadianone), K_2 (menaquinone) and K_3 (menadione). Vitamin K_1 and K_2 differ from K_3 in that they have a second side chain on the right ring of the molecule. Vitamin K_3 is a synthetic vitamin that is activated in the liver; vitamin K_1 is produced in plants, and vitamin K_2 by intestinal bacteria. The K vitamins are soluble in fats and insoluble in water, stable to heat but destroyed in acid and alkaline solutions. They are unstable to light and oxidizing agents.[205]

Raw milk, liver, kelp, other green plants, egg yolks and soybean oil (all in raw form) are also sources of vitamin K. A half cup of cooked spinach contains 275 percent of the RDA (recommended daily allowance) for vitamin K for adult men (80mcg) (the RDA for adult women is 60mcg); raw broccoli contains 165 percent the RDA per half cup; and a half cup of strawberries offers 20 percent. In addition, much study has been made of

---

[205] Sackheim, pages 432-433

cereal grasses and its vitamin K content (280mcg per 3.5 grams[206]) interwoven with other food factors, including beta carotene, amino acids, chlorophyll and a host of minerals. "In the 1930s and 1940s, before vitamin K could be easily synthesized, dehydrated cereal grasses were given before liver or gall-bladder surgery because it was the richest source of vitamin K available. Numerous medical studies reported excellent recoveries from this type of surgery when dehydrated cereal grass was administered...In addition, vitamin K has been used successfully for reducing excessive menstrual flow and cramps."[207] Further, green vegetables, particularly the cereal grasses (raw), are "our best sources of vitamin K. Although synthetic forms of this vitamin have been shown to be toxic when taken in excessive amounts, natural vitamin K (in whole foods) remains nontoxic, even in extremely high doses."[208]

Vitamin K serves as a cofactor for the processing of proteins required in the complex chain of reactions that regulates blood clotting. "One of these proteins is *prothrombin*, the inactive precursor of the enzyme that creates fibrin clots from fibrinogen. Vitamin K also assists in the synthesis of *osteocalcin*, a bone protein that forms the matrix for mineralization and bone building...Vitamin K is required for healing fractured bone and in the maintenance of normal bone...[and] may decrease calcium excretion and

---

[206] Seibold, page 51, citing: Kohler, G. 1953. The unidentified vitamins of grass and alfalfa. *Feedstuffs*, August 8, 1953; and Laboratory Analyses, September 6, 1989. Nutrition International, East Brunswick, NJ.

[207] ibid, page 60, citing: Rhoads, J. 1939. The relation of vitamin K to the hemorrhagic tendency in obstructive jaundice with a report on cerophyll as a source of vitamin K. *Surgery* 5:794-808; and Nutrition Search, Inc. 1984. *Nutrition Almanac.*, McGraw-Hill. New York.

[208] ibid, page 60, citing: Scott, M. 1986. *Nutrition of Humans and Selected Animal Species*. John Wiley and Sons. New York.

protect against osteoporosis."[209] Therefore, a deficiency of vitamin K points to a lack of prothrombin, resulting in a longer clotting time by the blood.

The relationship between vitamin K and the manufacture of bone proteins has led the American Society for Nutritional Sciences to proclaim the relationship between vitamin K status and skeletal health of the elderly. "If these findings turn out to be correct, they will open an exciting new area of research in the field of vitamin K metabolism."[210]

Without vitamin K, bones produce an abnormal protein that cannot bind to the mineral crystal deposits normally accumulating in the bones. The rate of synthesis of this protein is regulated by vitamin D.[211]

Vitamin K is also involved as a cofactor for oxidative phosphorylation reactions (the metabolic process of forming high energy phosphate bonds by introducing a phosphate group into an organic molecule—to create energy within the mitochondria of cells).

In the intestinal tract, vitamin K is synthesized by the presence of bacteria. For this reason, vitamin K deficiency may occur in cases of diarrhea. Vitamin K is absorbed from the small intestine with the help of bile. When bile fails to enter the small intestine, such as in obstructive jaundice or liver and/or gallbladder disease, vitamin K is not absorbed and deficiency may ensue. This condition leads to a tendency to bleed for a long period of time following injury (or surgery). In the occurrence of this problem in surgery, doctors may administer both bile and vitamin K to ensure blood coagulation.

---

[209] Ronzio, page 450.

[210] American Society for Nutritional Sciences, re: Suttie, J.W. (1992) Vitamin K and human nutrition. *J. Am. Diet. Assoc.* 92: 585-590 ; Suttie, J.W. (1993) Synthesis of vitamin K-dependent proteins. *FASEB* J. 7: 445-452 ; Booth, S.L., Pennington, J.A.T. & Sadowski, J.A. (1996) Food sources and dietary intakes of vitamin K-1 (phylloquinone) in the American diet: *J. Am. Diet. Assoc.* 96: 149-154.

[211] Whitney, page 262, re: Price, P.A., Role of vitamin-K dependent proteins in bone metabolism, *Annual Review of Nutrition* 8 (1988); 565-583.

One textbook on nutrition describes a possible scenario in which vitamin K deficiency may occur in the course of medical treatment: "A hospital [patient] with marginal vitamin K stores is given antibiotics to prevent or overcome infection and is fed a formula diet that does not include vitamin K. The antibiotics kill intestinal bacteria, and vitamin K stores are depleted. During surgery, the blood fails to clot normally, and the [patient] bleeds to death. The combination of antibiotics, unsupplemented formula diet, and surgery raises a warning flag and requires that clotting time be checked before surgery is performed. People taking sulfa drugs, which destroy intestinal bacteria, may also become deficient in vitamin K."[212] Antibiotic drugs are also known to destroy intestinal flora.

Because little of vitamin K is able to pass from mother to fetus during pregnancy, and since the infant gut is free of bacteria, vitamin K deficiency is most common in newborns. Breast milk is very low in vitamin K. It is now standard procedure to administer synthetic vitamin K by injection to newborns (as well as expectant mothers) to prevent hemorrhaging in the brain. Opponents of this procedure argue that there is a possibility for synthetic vitamin K to damage the liver of infants, or create allergic-type reactions. And some textbooks teach that vitamin K toxicity occurs only as a result of supplement overuse: "Excessive doses result in the clotting and breaking of blood cells. This releases the yellow pigment, bilirubin into the circulation, which can cause brain damage at high levels. The treatment for vitamin K toxicity is to give [the drug] dicumarol, which interferes with vitamin K activity and prevents blood from clotting. Vitamin K is one of the few vitamins that are regulated in supplements."[213] Medical sources claim that occurrences of vitamin K toxicity from overdose in infants are rare.

Standard medical advice warns against the intake of green, leafy vegetables and its vitamin K factors in cases of stroke and heart attack which is feared

---

[212] ibid.
[213] Smolin, page 274.

caused by blood clotting. Following the clot, according to medical resources, the flow of blood through the vessels is obstructed, thus depriving the brain/heart of oxygen and nutrients. However, there are a few doctors who argue that neither stroke nor heart attack is *caused* by clotting, but rather that blood clotting is instead the result blood leakage through damaged/cracked vessels. In consideration of this, there is a controversy as to the potential disaster latent in prescribing anti-coagulation drugs without concern for repairing already damaged and leaking blood vessels, because hemorrhaging (bleeding to death) is a distinct possibility when the blood is unable to clot.

STANDARDIZATION IN HERBAL
& FOOD SUPPLEMENTS

One of the enigmas of nature is that, as with human beings, no two foods are the same. They may compare in color, size, shape and species, yet the nutrient values of two similar foods are guaranteed to vary. One carrot may be ten times as rich in carotenes than another. And an echinacea plant growing near a railroad track in Kentucky may contain more vitamin A precursors than an echinacea plant growing in an environment-controlled greenhouse at a leading university. With the popularity of herbs—a rediscovery of their healing powers and nutrient value from ancient medical practice—supplement manufacturers have become frustrated over the variations in the efficacy and potency of herbal ingredients. So, to ensure predictability, man once again has set out to improve nature in a practice now known as "standardization."

Standardization is a blending together of natural healthcare and scientific intervention. The end result is an unnatural creation: herbs mixed with synthetic or fractionated constituents—usually vitamins and flavonoids. Enough has been stated about the imbalances arriving out of fractionated and synthetic substances without reiteration here. When it comes to herbal medicine, the caveat "buyer beware" continues in full effect.

Perhaps the most overlooked issue regarding standardization of herbs is that there is more value to herbs than vitamins alone. For many herbalists, vitamins are very low on the list of herbal functions, making standardization an exercise in "missing the point." Rather than looking to herbs as sources of bioflavonoids, herbalists generally use herbs for their effects—warming, cooling, heating, drying, moisturizing, tonifying, etc. Few herbalists would argue that many of the benefits of herbs are not even scientifically measurable owing to their energetic effects rather than their nutrient effects.

Although it is now common to infuse herbal supplements with synthetic and isolated vitamins and flavonoids, we have no way of calculating how this practice interferes with the other functions and usages of herbal preparations.

ANTIOXIDANTS & FREE RADICALS

The very word "antioxidant" has only recently entered our vocabulary to describe substances protecting the body from destruction by "free radicals." However, the knowledge of oxygen's (or air's) potential to alter and damage foods is not especially new. For some time, scientists have been aware of the molecular changes in foods due to the exposure of certain fats (like butter and oil) to air. This awareness eventually led to mandatory refrigeration and improved food packaging.[214] The fear of impaired health due to exogenous assault from the environment and consumption of nonfood substances has dramatically boosted the fame and fortune associated with the now-burgeoning antioxidant supplement market.

Generally speaking, antioxidants are considered to be the vitamins A, C and E, plus the minerals selenium, copper, zinc and manganese. In whole foods, antioxidants team up with other food constituents, including other vitamins and enzymes (for example, vitamin E with selenium, or vitamin C with vitamin E). Antioxidant compounds found in foods also include bioflavonoids, coenzyme Q10 (generally in fish, nuts and lean meats); and sulfur-containing amino acids.

In the drama of life, free radicals are the villains, while antioxidants are the heroes in the white hats. Oxygen is the fought-over prize. Free radicals are highly reactive oxygen fragments created by cellular function and metabolism. They lack electrons and attempt to steal them from other molecules to regroup. This natural process is referred to as *oxidation*. Free

---

[214] McCarrison, M.D., Robert, *Studies in Deficiency Disease,* Henry Frowde and Hodder & Stoughton, London, 1921.

radicals include the superoxide radical, the hydroxyl radical and hydrogen peroxide. A certain level of free radicals is essential for good health, as they are involved in mechanisms such as fighting infection and in the contraction of smooth muscles in the blood vessels.

Cells have a number of ways of dealing with excess free radicals, including the use of enzyme systems and specific antioxidants. Antioxidants are substances which surrender their own electrons easily for the purpose of neutralizing oxidants, including free radicals. If the body becomes overwhelmed with free radicals, the body's own antioxidants may not be enough to offer protection. The result is that free radicals stabilize themselves by taking electrons from chemically stable compounds, often causing the generation of more free radicals which react further with other compounds, causing yet more damage. These split-second chain reactions spread throughout the body, attacking vulnerable sites in the cells and causing damage that can result in chronic disease through destruction of living tissue.

Exogenous (external) assaults on the body's biochemistry by now-common poisons such as cigarette smoke [both passive and active], heavy metals such as cadmium, mercury and lead, pesticide and synthetic fertilizer ingestion, toxic fumes and inhalants, air and water pollution, radioactive particles, industrial and automotive waste, radiation and ultraviolet light lead to free radical damage. Certain vitamins (mentioned above) tend to place themselves into the free radical chain to protect the body. These vitamins are altered in sacrifice to the body's cells that would have otherwise taken place. Further, antioxidants are said to interact to protect one another. Vitamin C, for instance is known to protect a damaged vitamin E molecule by converting it back to its antioxidant status. Vitamin C is then likewise saved by another antioxidant such as glutathione. Vitamin E, on the other hand, is known to protect the oxidation of vitamin A and unsaturated fatty acids.[215] This is one of the reasons why many supplement

---

[215] Sackheim, page 432.

manufacturers add ascorbic acid and mixed tocopherols to their ingredients—to protect the other vitamins and essential fatty acids in the formula itself. Even more importantly, this is one of the reasons nature provides **a complement of vitamins, minerals, enzymes, coenzymes, trace minerals, essential fatty acids and amino acids in whole foods.** This complement of co-constituents is, of course, absent in fractionated and synthetic supplements.

The body produces several enzymes, including *superoxide dismutase* (SOD), catalase and glutathione peroxidase that neutralize many types of free radicals. Taking supplements of these enzymes may or may not be effective, depending on absorption, as well as the presence of specific mineral-activators that act as building blocks. Needed in the diet, then, are manganese, zinc and copper for SOD, and selenium for glutathione peroxidase.[216] Natural, whole foods and whole food supplements contain **both the antioxidant and the activators and synergists needed for optimum function.**

Free radicals are known to freely attack various bodily systems, including DNA (leading to cancer and abnormal cellular mutation); blood fats leading to CVD (cardiovascular diseases); cholesterol; cellular enzymes; the mitochondria of cells (the energy-producing powerhouse of cells); nerves; the eye and its lens (connected to macular degeneration and cataracts); joints and the musculoskeletal system (as in gout and arthritis); the respiratory system (as in asthma and other pulmonary-related diseases); reproductive and hormonal systems; and possibly the linings of tissues to cause artery, stomach, intestinal and skin damage. Free radicals are also suspected of causing damage to major organs such as the kidneys, adrenal glands and liver.

Antioxidant research, as reported in the *Annals of Internal Medicine*, is considering that there may be more to antioxidants at work in providing health and prevention that should not be overlooked. In addition to providing antioxidant benefits, some studies have shown that the so-called

---

[216] Lininger, page 267.

"antioxidant" vitamins may also work to preserve endothelial [as well as epithelial] cell function, affect hemostasis [the arrest of bleeding], and lower LDL cholesterol levels and blood pressure.[217]

Detecting free radicals

Because there is no way to directly detect free radical production in humans, indirect methods have been developed. Basically these methods rely on the breakdown products of lipid peroxidation, such as conjugated diene (unsaturated hydrocarbons), malondialdehyde (MDA), and

---

[217] *Annals of Internal Medicine*: Online report 1999. "The Antioxidant Vitamins and Cardiovascular Disease A Critical Review of Epidemiologic and Clinical Trial Data," Prabhat Jha, MD, DPhil; Marcus Flather, MBBS, MRCP; Eva Lonn, MD, FRCPC; Michael Farkouh, MD, FRCPC; and Salim Yusuf, DPhil, FRCP, citing: Reaven PD, Khouw A, Beltz WF, Parthasarathy S, WitztumJL. Effect of dietary antioxidant combinations in humans.Protection of LDL by vitamin E but not by beta-carotene. *ArteriosclerThromb.* 1993;13:590-600; Sato K, Niki E, Shimasaki H. Free radical-mediatedchain oxidation of low density lipoproteins and its synergistic inhibition by vitamin E and vitamin C. *Arch Biochem Biophys.* 1990;279:402-5.; Willett WC, Stampfer MJ, Underwood BA, Taylor JO, HennekensCH. Vitamins A, E, and carotene: effects of supplementation on their plasma levels. *Am J Clin Nutr.* 1983;38:559-66; *Green J.* Interrelationships between vitamin E and other vitamins and the ubiquinones. *Vitam Horm.* 1962;20:485-94; Farrell PM, Bieri JG. Megavitamin E supplementation in man. *Am J Clin Nutr.* 1975;28:1381-6; Keaney JF Jr, Gaziano JM, Xu A, Frei B, Curran-CelentanoJ, Shwaery GT, et al. Dietary antioxidants preserve endothelium-dependent vessel relaxation in cholesterol-fed rabbits. *Proc Natl Acad Sci,* U S A. 1993;90:11880-4; Khaw KT, Woodhouse P. Interrelation of vitamin C, infection,haemostatic factors, and cardiovascular disease. *BMJ.* 1995;310:1559-63; Trout DL. Vitamin C and cardiovascular risk factors.*Am J Clin Nutr.* 1991;53:322S-5S; Jacques PF. Effects of vitamin C on high-density lipoprotein cholesterol and blood pressure. *J Am Coll Nutr.* 1992;11:139-44; Stamler J, Ruth KJ, Liu K, Shekkele RB. Dietary antioxidant sand blood pressure change in the western electric study [Abstract].34th Annual Conference on Cardiovascular Disease Epidemiology and Prevention. Tampa, Florida; 1993.

hydrocarbons. Measurement of malondialdehyde and conjugated dienes in the blood or urine and the assessment of hydrocarbon production by measurement of expired pentane provide evidence of lipid peroxidation. Malondialdehyde is most commonly measured by its reaction with thiobarbituric acid, which generates thiobarbituric acid reactive substances (TBARS). These methods, however, have been criticized for not representing an accurate measure of lipid peroxidation. Because lipid peroxidation can occur in all tissues, it is argued that blood levels of peroxidation products or expired pentane can provide no information on *where* lipid peroxidation is occurring. Furthermore, expired pentane can reflect flushing of hydrocarbons from adipose tissue, and many natural compounds *other than lipids* can produce TBARS.

Another approach to oxidation and antioxidant study is to assess blood levels of vitamins E (tocopherol), C, and A. But, because no one of these measures provides an accurate assessment of lipid peroxidation or antioxidant status, studies have incorporated several assessments. "Until more valid techniques are developed, our knowledge of free radical generation, oxidative stress, and antioxidant status is limited."[218] However difficult to assess in the human biochemistry, there seems to be little

---

[218] Clarkson, Ph.D.,Priscilla M., "Antioxidants: What are They and What Role Do They Play in Physical Activity and Health? " (Abstract from NIH Workshop:The Role of Dietary Supplements for Physically Active People), HealthWorld Online, March, 2000, re: Alessio HM. Exercise-induced oxidative stress. *Med Sci Sports Exerc* 1993;25:218-24; Bendich A. Exercise and free radicals: effects of antioxidant vitamins. *Med Sport Sci* 1991;32:59-78; Clarkson PM. Antioxidants and physical performance. *Clin Rev Food Sci Nutr* 1995;35:131 41; Clarkson PM. Micronutrients and exercise: anti-oxidants and minerals. J *Sports Sci* 1995;13:SII-S24; Dekkers JC, van Doornen LJP, Kemper HCG. The role of antioxidant vitamins and enzymes in the prevention of exercise-induced muscle damage. *Sports Med* 1996;21:213-38; Goldfarb AH. Antioxidants: role of supplementation to prevent exercise-induced oxidative stress. *Med Sci Sports Exerc* 1993;25:232-6; Sjodin B. Hellsten Westing Y. Apple FS. Biochemical mechanisms for oxygen free radical formation during exercise. *Sports Med* 1990;10:236-54.

argument among researchers of the damages of oxidation as well as the beneficial activity of antioxidants.

Whole Foods Offer Antioxidant Protection from More Than Just One Isolated Vitamin or Flavonoid...

One group of researchers at the Agricultural Research Service (ARS), led by Dr. Ron Prior at the Jean Mayer USDA Human Nutrition Research Center on Aging at Tufts in Boston, has taken a close look at antioxidants by assaying protective effects of fruits and vegetables. This group is finding that blueberries, strawberries, red bell peppers, Concord grapes, and beets—along with several deep-green vegetables—are "workhorses at disarming free radicals, at least in the test tube. Recent large clinical trials have focused on specific antioxidant compounds in fruits and vegetables, such as beta carotene, vitamin C, or vitamin E. But 'fruits and vegetables have many other antioxidant compounds,' says Prior. 'Much of the protection they confer against cancer, heart disease, and stroke may be from compounds other than these vitamins.'"[219] Prior and his colleagues, Drs. Guohua Cao, Hong Wang and Emin Sofic, work to determine the total antioxidant capacity of specific fruits and vegetables using a special chemical assay. Prior's group ran the assay for total antioxidant capacity on more than a dozen commonly eaten fruits, five fruit juices, and more than a score of vegetables and other foods. They also tested green and black teas. Scoring highest among fruits and juices tested were blueberries, strawberries, and grape juice.

> Three and one-half ounces of blueberries—about two-thirds of a cup worth—disarmed as many peroxyl radicals as 1,773 International Units (IU) of vitamin E or 1,270mg of vitamin C did. Strawberries were more than half as potent as blueberries. Plums scored third, having nearly two-thirds the total antioxidant

---

[219] McBride

capacity of strawberries. Among the 22 vegetables assayed, kale led the bunch with a total antioxidant capacity a little above that of strawberries, followed by spinach with about the same potency as plums. Three and one-half ounces of kale—an easily edible portion—disarmed as many free radicals as 837 IU of vitamin E or 599 mg of vitamin C did. Total antioxidant capacity of kale was about twice as potent as beets and broccoli flowers, 8 to 9 times more potent than carrots and string beans, and 29 to 35 times more potent than celery and cucumber.[220]

Testing strawberries and all of their selected vegetables against two other oxidizing agents generated via normal metabolism—the hydroxyl radical and copper ions, the Boston researchers came to an interesting conclusion regarding the complex properties of whole foods. In earlier studies, Dr. Cao discovered "that vitamins C and E can actually be turncoats while in the company of transition metals—such as copper or iron ions—and become oxidizing agents themselves. **Such was not the case when the whole fruit or vegetable** extract was pitted against copper ions, Cao reported.

"Whole fruits and vegetables contain a mixture of natural antioxidants that can protect the vulnerable compounds." Which of these compounds get absorbed by the body and increase protection from oxidative stress or improve health in some other fashion? The researchers are currently conducting studies on rodents to get some preliminary answers. "If the animal studies produce positive results," says Prior, "it gives us a measure of **the quality of foods other than the common nutrients bio-medical science has been looking at.**"[221]

---

220 Ibid.
221 Ibid.

Antioxidants & Aging

Much antioxidant study is now involved in the fight against aging—a seemingly inevitable stage of life. In addition to the slow-down of metabolic processes that occur with aging, it is now believed that premature aging and rapid aging may be due to the accumulation of various adverse changes in cells and tissues that increase the risk of death.

Evidence is growing that free radicals are an underlying cause of aging as the biological markers of the process are the same as those caused by free radical damage. As the mitochondria are where most of the oxygen reactions in the cell occur, they may be the most susceptible to damage by free radicals. It has been suggested that the rate of damage, and therefore aging, in mitochondria may determine how long a person lives. The ability of antioxidants to reduce this damage explains their possible role in slowing the aging process. Research into chemicals which could slow the damage to mitochondria without decreasing energy production is in the early stages but it is expected to increase. Due to their effects on mitochondria and other elements such as cell membranes and genetic material, free radicals may aggravate the breakdown and sagging of tissues and deterioration of bodily organs involved in the aging process. Many diseases commonly associated with aging, including cancer, heart disease and psychological disorders, appear to be prevented or improved by increasing intake of antioxidants. High levels of antioxidants also increase the effectiveness of the immune system, making older people less susceptible to life-threatening infections.[222]

Experiments with aging animals show that the effectiveness of the body's antioxidant system decreases with age, possibly because of reduced dietary intake, absorption and/or increased nutrient needs. A steady supply of

---

[222] *Vitamin Update*, Bookman Press online, 1998..

antioxidant vitamins and minerals is hoped to enhance the body's natural defense mechanisms and improve the quality and length of life.[223]

Because the modern-day diet is typically mostly devoid of (or severely lacking in) real, whole and live foods, most Westerners fail to consume antioxidant foods that offer substantial protection. Processed and heated (pasteurized and cooked) foods contain no live food complexes with their vitamin, mineral, enzyme and amino acids fully intact.

One study published by Johns Hopkins University in Baltimore shows that diets high in fruit and vegetables (whole foods) can increase the antioxidant capacity of the blood. During the study, involving 123 people over a period of eleven weeks, "researchers examined the effects of three diets on oxidative processes in cells. One group ate a high fat, low fruit and vegetable diet, the second group ate a low fat, high fruit and vegetable diet and the third group ate a high fat, high fruit and vegetable diet. When researchers measured breath *ethane* production, a marker for cellular oxidative processes, they found that this was reduced in those whose diets were high in fruit and vegetables. Resistance to oxidative damage also increased in those participants."[224]

Phytochemical Research Laboratory program officer Ronald Prior, Ph.D., has worked extensively to identify the antioxidant capacity of foods. Measuring the total antioxidant capacity of specific biological samples, the laboratory's researchers study the total antioxidant activity of foods as well as animal tissues and human blood to uncover the degree of protection provided by antioxidants against hydroxyl or peroxyl radicals. One study, of eight healthy elderly women's serum, following the consumption of meals known to have either high or low *oxygen radical absorbance capacities* (ORAC), produced "interesting results." ORAC "increased significantly after consumption of any meal. Serum ORAC increased by a greater amount than control after a single meal supplemented with strawberry

---

[223] ibid.
[224] *Circulation* 1998;98:2390-95.

extract or spinach extract or red wine with the alcohol removed or a single dose of 1250 mg Vitamin C."[225] Dr. Prior reports,

> We hypothesize that endogenous antioxidant activity increases after the consumption of any meal either to prepare for, or in reaction to, the rise in reactive oxygen species (ROS) due to increased metabolic activity. Consumption of meals high in antioxidants supplements the endogenous antioxidant activity increase, [thereby] causing the observed greater ORAC increase. Since an increase in serum ORAC similar to that after strawberry and spinach treatments was also noted after a single 1250 mg dose of Vitamin C, it was concluded that those **doses of strawberry and spinach extracts produce an antioxidant response equivalent to a 1250 mg dose of Vitamin C.**[226]

Ingestion of vitamin C as a synthetic (sold as ascorbic acid, ester C, etc.), despite all of its hooplah as an antioxidant, is missing the synergists (including bioflavnoids, enzymes, etc.) to be found in whole foods. The USDA's Agricultural Research Services shows that whole foods not only provide adequate antioxidant value, but much more than vitamin C alone can offer. Researchers concluded: "Eating a half pound of strawberries or spinach can be just as effective as taking a large dose of vitamin C in helping the human body defuse oxygen radicals that can damage cells. Next, they wanted to find out whether those protective compounds could be absorbed by the human body in sufficient amounts to boost the blood's antioxidant profile. They analyzed the blood of eight women in their 60s and 70s before and after eating five test meals. Each woman first ate a control meal with a low antioxidant content. Then, over the course of two

---

225 Prior, Ph.D., Ronald L., "Bioavailability and Health Benefits of Phytochemicals in Fruits and Vegetables," Phytochemical Research Laboratory, 1999.

226 ibid.

months, the researchers added either a strawberry extract, a spinach extract, red wine or 1,250 milligrams of vitamin C to the control meal. The strawberry and spinach extracts were consumed as drinks having the equivalent of 8 to 10 ounces of the produce."[227]

> Simply eating the control meal increased the antioxidants circulating in the women's blood up to 10 percent. The strawberry and spinach extracts boosted the antioxidant capacity another 20 percent. That's as much protection as the women got from taking the vitamin C. Red wine was somewhat less effective, boosting antioxidant capacity by 15 percent above the control level. Some but not all of the antioxidant boost was due to vitamin C and uric acid—an antioxidant made by the body, the researchers found. They conclude that other antioxidants—probably polyphenols—are being absorbed from the **fruits and vegetables**.[228]

Although the general public and the healthcare industry alike tend to gravitate to the use of antioxidant supplements in the form of isolates and synthetics for protection against free radicals, certain foods have shown to offer not only a great supply of antioxidants, but also a host of synergists needed as cofactors for myriad biochemical functions. Now many of these plant food nutrients are being referred to as *phytochemicals* (also, and more accurately, *phytonutrients*), and include dark, green leafy vegetables high in chlorophyll and vitamin A precursors (especially beta carotene), flavonoids, and trace minerals. Specific components of foods such as lutein (used especially in macular degeneration studies), specific B vitamins, cysteine, lycopene (used in cancer studies), and coenzyme Q10 (also called ubiquinone and used in heart research and studies on energy production within the cell), are being applauded for their antioxidant capabilities.[229] Coenzyme Q10, as shown in

---

227 Prior, Ph.D., Ronald L and Cao, Dr. Guohua, *USDA Human Nutrition Research Center on Aging at Tufts, Boston, MA; USDA Agricultural Research Service, July 1997*
228 ibid.
229 Lininger, page 267.

double-blind research, may play a healthful role against congestive heart failure.[230] Several herbs that stand out in their antioxidant capacity include cayenne, garlic, turmeric, ginkgo biloba, pine bark, grape seed, ginger and bilberry.

Thanks to a great deal of research being performed in the dwindling rainforests of South and Central America by devoted scientists such as James Duke, Ph.D. and Leslie Taylor, N.D. (to name only two) more discoveries of valuable herbs and exotic foods—fruits, berries, barks, nuts, seeds and roots—are being made.

Antioxidants in the Mediterranean Diet

French researchers report that the typical Mediterranean diet (replete with antioxidant foods) appears to protect against heart disease. Analysis of the diets of more than 600 patients participating in the Lyon Heart Study has shown that those who ate large amounts of fish, fruit, vegetables, bread, wine and monounsaturated oils had a reduced risk of heart disease. The researchers compared fatal and nonfatal heart attack occurrences in two groups: those eating a typical Western diet (control group) and those eating a Mediterranean diet. There were 59 coronary events in the control group and 14 in the Mediterranean diet group. Researchers believe that these effects are due to the higher levels of antioxidant vitamins and omega-3-fatty acids in Mediterranean diets.[231]

---

[230] Lininger, page 283, re: Mortensen SA, Vadhanavikit S, Baandrup U, Folkers K. Long-term coenzyme Q10 therapy: a major advance in the management of resistant myocardial failure. *Drug Exptl Clin Res*, 1985; 11: 581-93; and Morisco C, Trimarco B, Condorelli M. Effect of coenzyme Q10 in patients with congestive heart failure: a long-term multicenter randomized study. *Clin Invest* 1993; 71: S134-136.

[231] *Journal of the American College of Cardiology* 1996: 28 from *Vitamin News*, December 1996.

Antioxidants and Athletics

Researchers at California State University, as reported at the 5th Annual Meeting of the Oxygen Society, focused on the antioxidant properties of pine bark and its promise to improve exercise endurance. Pine bark extracts were used in a study involving 24 male and female athletes, aged from 15 to 30. The report stated, "Half of the participants received a placebo for 30 days followed by 30 days of pine bark, while the other half received pine bark first. Researchers then tested oxygen consumption and time to exhaustion during exercise in the athletes. The results showed that endurance improved by nearly 30 percent in the group that received pine bark first compared to 14 percent in those who received placebo. Pine bark contains compounds known as *proanthocyanidins*, which have antioxidant effects."[232]

Additional studies of antioxidants are being conducted with regard to exercise pertaining to professional and hard-training amateurs, as well as "weekend athletes." Studying the role of antioxidants in physical activity, Priscilla M. Clarkson, Ph.D. writes,

> Certain highly reactive chemical species called free radicals increase during exercise. Free radicals contain one or more unpaired electrons in their outer orbit that allows them to attack cellular components. During oxidative metabolism, most of the consumed oxygen ends up bound to hydrogen, forming water. Because this process is not 100 percent effective, 4-5 percent of the oxygen is not completely reduced and forms free radicals which, in turn, lead to other harmful oxidation products. When free radicals attack cellular membranes, a chain of reactions called lipid peroxidation produces additional damage. Thus, as oxygen consumption is increased during exercise, there will be a

---

[232] 5th Annual Meeting of the Oxygen Society, Reuters.

concomitant increase in free radicals and lipid peroxidation in skeletal muscle cells.

Exercise can also generate free radicals by other means, including (1) increased intake of oxygen which itself is a diradical, (2) increased amounts of epinephrine and other catecholamines that produce oxygen radicals when they are metabolically inactivated, (3) production of lactic acid that can convert a weakly damaging free radical (superoxide) into a (4) response to membranes and an increase in macrophages and white blood cells in damaged muscle.[233]

Clark concludes that there is no conclusive evidence showing the exact amounts of antioxidants needed to benefit persons subjected to vigorous training and exercise. She writes,

Popular belief is that high doses of vitamins C, E, and beta carotene are not harmful. However, in recent years concern has arisen over the long-term use of megadoses of selected nutrients. **When one considers that the body operates on a finely tuned homeostasis, it would appear that megadoses of any nutrient could upset the delicate balance. Moreover, it may take a long time before the resulting negative effects are evident.**

Many sports nutritionists recommend that adequate amounts of antioxidants be obtained from the diet, and that athletes should make intelligent food choices. As an 'insurance policy,' athletes could be encouraged to take a multivitamin/mineral supplement containing no more than the recommended dietary allowance (RDA). In contrast, other experts believe that there is sufficient information to suggest that athletes supplement their diets with antioxidants in excess of the RDA. Some have suggested that it borders on malpractice not to recommend antioxidant supplements to

---

[233] Clarkson

athletes. Although the issue of whether to supplement with antioxidants and how much to supplement remains unresolved, what is clear is **the importance of ingesting foods rich in antioxidants** for those who exercise regularly as well as those who exercise on occasion."[234]

Antioxidant Fad

As with any other product that attracts the input of many individuals and corporations who stand to gain by excessive promotion, promises and anecdotal testimonials, antioxidants have risen to the top of the charts as the substances we've just "gotta have." Therefore, they have joined the ranks of a wide array of vitamins, minerals, amino acids and herbs promoted in fad-like fashion, with the greatest selling point being the fear of death and disease by a very real assault of pollutants and chemicals that human civilization has never had to deal with. Like vitamins and the rest, antioxidants are being extracted out of their original food complexes (isolated/fractionated) and tableted or encapsulated for supplementation. Because studies are so inconclusive about appropriate dosages, or even the necessity for supplementation, the safest bet is to consume antioxidants either in whole, natural food form or within whole food supplements.

---

[234] ibid.

Bio-Individuality, Modern Science & Natural Solutions

We are all different, which is why we are called "individuals." Yet the shotgun approach to natural healthcare seems to be the standard among consumers, with the prevailing but misguided philosophy of "It's good for me, so it must be good for you too." What makes one person different from the next? The human body, mind and emotions are extremely complex. As such, when a patient comes to the doctor for care, the doctor is seeing only the tip of the iceberg. This is why native healers, such as traditional Chinese or Native American doctors, often insisted on living with their patients for a couple of weeks or more prior to suggesting any form of treatment. Not only does a patient have symptoms and diseases to consider, but also genetics, daily diet, childhood illnesses, emotional trauma, race, anatomical peculiarities, tolerances, age, sex, climate, tobacco and alcohol use, sexual activity, sanitary habits, exercise or lack thereof, hobbies (exposure to glues, resins, dust, gasoline, etc.), religious beliefs, innate fears, stress factors, particular thinking processes, location and environment of residence (urban, suburban, noise, pollution, stress, dampness, dryness, etc.) digestive status, sleep problems, drug usage (legal and illegal), temperament, metabolism, attitude, intellect and tastes. The variables, combinations and interrelationships are staggering.

Research findings are continually affected by the aforementioned factors of the complexities of human beings—one great argument against using a "one size fits all" mentality for supplement and drug usage, despite promising studies.

154

Moreover, it is common for studies to have potentially important methodological problems that limit their interpretation, as evidenced by a team of medical doctors involved in the study "The Antioxidant Vitamins and Cardiovascular Disease: A Critical Review of Epidemiologic and Clinical Trial Data." While the supplements in this particular study may at first seem to hold promise against cardiovascular disease, researchers were careful to note that people who take antioxidants may also tend to be *more health conscious than those who do not*, leaving researchers to wonder whether the use of supplements is only a common-denominator among already healthier individuals, and not that the supplements themselves should take the credit for the health of their users. Researchers noted

...lifestyle and dietary patterns probably differ significantly between persons who use and do not use antioxidant vitamins. For example, in four of the larger studies...persons using antioxidant vitamins were, on aggregate and in relative percentages, 24% less likely to be current smokers, 29% more likely to exercise regularly, and 10% less likely to have hypertension than persons who did not use the vitamins. Persons using antioxidant vitamins also consumed less alcohol. These findings suggest that persons using antioxidant vitamins may have other health and lifestyle behaviors that reduce their risk for cardiovascular disease. The absolute difference in these behaviors is not large enough to significantly alter the risk reductions seen for vitamin E or vitamin C intake; in addition, these differences have been considered in most of the cohort studies we examined, either by stratification or adjustment in statistical models. However, such adjustment may be unreliable if these other variables were measured poorly (such as a single unreliable blood pressure reading). Moreover, it is impossible to adjust for unmeasured health behaviors that probably exist, given the more healthy profile of persons using antioxidant vitamins.[235]

Astute and experienced healthcare practitioners have been witness to many patients' exclamations of the wonders of their supplements in arresting all sorts of symptoms while pondering that perhaps a lifestyle change had more to do with profound health benefits than just the supplements. For example, a patient complaining of monthly migraine headaches may pick up a bottle of feverfew and begin using it religiously. During the next office visit she tells her doctor that her headaches are gone, thanks to the feverfew. But she forgets to mention that she got a new job and her marital problems were all worked out or that she gave up foods with artificial ingredients due to a magazine article she read—all possible causes of the headaches in the first place. In another example, there was man who suffered terribly all winter from eczema-type rashes all over his arms and legs and went from doctor to doctor looking for relief. He tried a variety of supplements—herbs, vitamins and essential fatty acids—and lotions with no relief. Then one day, when the weather turned warmer, the man noticed that his skin eruptions went away. To make a long story short, the man discovered that his skin rashes were caused from the woolen suit he was wearing during the cooler times of the year. After his rash disappeared, as an experiment, he wore his woolen pants again, and within a day the rash reappeared. He stopped wearing wool and the problem never returned. If the man had merely stopped wearing his woolen suit without ever making the cause-and-effect connection, then his recovery could have been attributed to lifestyle change, a miracle or one of the supplements he began taking. Such is the complexity of life and health.

---

235 *Annals of Internal Medicine*. Online report 1999. "The Antioxidant Vitamins and Cardiovascular Disease A Critical Review of Epidemiologic and Clinical Trial Data. Prabhat Jha, MD, et.al.

Many factors relative to human health, healing, energy and vitality are completely intangible, such as emotions and thinking processes, yet they influence the overall health as much as the daily diet. Some doctors will argue that emotions and mindset have a greater impact on health than any other factor. Headaches, ulcers, muscle tension, bowel irregularities, blurred vision, stroke, cardiac arrest and skin rashes have been known to manifest from emotional and mental problems. To date, the exact effects such emotions will have on health remain real but unpredictable. To complicate all of this, the body, mind and emotions change day to day, season to season, and year to year, and even with weather patterns. For this reason, traditional Chinese medicine has based its prescriptions and advice not on symptoms, isolated complaints or scientific studies of the efficacy of pharmacological agents, but rather on *symptom complexes*—a complex assessment of an array of symptoms that tend to create an overall picture of health. This takes a lot of work, research, experience and dedication to the patient—unheard of in today's fast-paced, magic bullet society.

In consideration of bioindividuality, to suggest that 10 grams of vitamin C per day is good for everyone, or that there's a cure for all cancers, or everyone needs colloidal minerals, or everyone benefits from fluoride in the water, is a dangerous, speculative and unscientific generalization. And so it is unwise to embrace every vitamin and drug fad that becomes en vogue year after year.

With enough marketing hype, as a society, we witness a stream of outrageous promises claiming that every new fad product is a panacea for all of our ills. And everyone starts to give advice on how to cure one another's ills. This has never been so evident than in the case of Ritalin, the drug most prescribed for hyperactivity in children. Parents with young school children can testify to the fact that teachers and other school officials (who are not medical authorities or doctors or nurses) have begun recommending Ritalin for behavior problems as if this drug were no more potent than the chemicalized chocolate chip cookies they use as treats for good behavior.

The resolution of hyperactivity, as with other health conditions, begs to be conveniently addressed with drugs rather than looking into the complexity of other factors that may be involved in the problem. For instance, some researchers such as Albert Burgstahler, Ph.D. (Harvard University, Organic Chemistry), point to the damaging effects of fluoride on human biochemistry as a possible cause of ADD (attention deficit disorder). Burgstahler shows that one of the most notable effects of fluoride is impaired thyroid function, thus leading to hyperactivity in children and hypoactivity in adults.[236] Other factors (one or a combination of two or more) contributing to hyperactivity may include overstimulation, ingestion of refined sugars, deficiency in B complex vitamins, mineral deficiencies, reactions to food chemicals in processed foods, learning disabilities, ingestion of soda pop, and the need for eyeglasses, nutritional deficiencies, and our electronic cyberworld that has outpaced the tedium of school work, to name a few. Rarely are all of the possible causative factors thoroughly exhausted before resorting to drug use because to do so demands an investment in time and observation.[237]

Like popular drugs, supplements of isolated vitamins, minerals, enzymes, and amino acids are also misused. Diet and lifestyle should be the doctor's first consideration prior to supplementation even with whole food supplements. Many health complaints disappear by fasting, radically changing to a raw food detox diet, moving out of a polluted environment, or learning to cope with stress. None of these solutions involve the ingestion of any supplement, drug or herbal extract.

In a country where more is better, and the quicker the results, the better served, we have a dilemma that crosses the boundary from healthcare to conscience. Modern medicine is theoretically founded on the Hippocratic

---

[236] *Acres, USA,* "The Fluoride Menace," March 2000.

[237] An excellent review of Ritalin is discussed in *The Myth of the A.D.D. Child* by Thomas Armstrong, Ph.D., Penguin Books, 1995.

Oath upon which the doctor agrees to "first do no harm." This may be interpreted as a caution to be careful—to act with care for the patient. With the conflicting reports on the efficacy and safety and toxicity of fractionated and synthetic supplementation, certainly care must be the first priority. Because the body is so wondrously complex, there remains a doubt as to whether it can be simply treated with the use of isolates without creating biochemical imbalances and toxicity of unforeseen magnitude. Further, regarding synthetic vitamins, the naturalist may argue that no synthetic, unnatural substance has any place or use in the human body. Thus is formed the argument between chemistry vs. biochemistry.

Ruth Kava, Ph.D., Director of Nutrition, American Council on Science and Health, explains: Vitamins and minerals, frequently "used in pharmacological doses (doses much larger than could be obtained from foods)," are not monitored for their effects to any great degree because they are generally accepted to be safe. "Thus, these chemicals (**vitamins and minerals are chemicals**) may be sold without prior certification that they are either safe or effective for the purposes for which people buy them, and without scientifically established dosage levels for particular purposes."[238] "Those who do not support the widespread use of dietary supplements for either insurance or prevention are concerned about two aspects of the use of such products: safety and effectiveness…'Safe' does not mean completely safe for everyone under all possible circumstances, however."[239]

On the other end of the spectrum from the vitamin advocates, researchers studying the Paleolithic diets of our human ancestors are pointing out that the most primal biochemical and physiological needs of the body are to be found in natural, whole and unaltered foods. Some call

---

[238] ibid.
[239] Kava, Ph.D., R.D., Ruth, *Vitamins & Minerals, Does the Epidemiologic Evidence Justify General Supplementation?*, 2nd Ed., American Council on Scienceand Health, Inc., February 2000

such findings science, while others label them common sense, because natural, whole, raw and unprocessed foods contain a complexity of nutrients that work harmoniously with the complexity of the human organism. Science's departure from nature (and nature's innate intelligence to create balance and feed all of the living organisms on earth) is in defiance not only of common sense, but also the essence of biology—a science in itself. Today's medical and scientific approach can only be related to Dr. Seuss' Cat in the Hat metaphor, wherein theoretical solutions lead to unseen problems which then create a problematic chain of events of unseen magnitude and predictability.

The modern, Western-world diet in our so-called "advanced" countries is based on convenience, taste and economics, while, in contrast, the biochemistry of the body is based on nutrient requirements found only in natural foods. This makes modern man and woman in conflict with themselves, leading to the appalling disease rate that we have in modern societies. Despite all the drugs, vitamins, creature comforts, technological innovations and advanced food processing methodology (all unnatural), modern society remains plagued with diseases that continue out of control—cancer, tuberculosis, asthma, dental carries, diabetes, cardiovascular disease, arthritis and more. Ignored and swept under the rug are causative factors of disease that include environmental toxins, pesticide use, fluoride and chlorine additives, plastic degassing, nuclear waste, genetic engineering, mental and emotional stress, the overconsumption of drugs, and ubiquitous pollution of air, water and land. The return to nature has never been more in demand for the salvation of humankind, the plant and animal kingdoms and the earth itself.

Unnatural, synthetic and short-cut solutions have been proven non-options for a diseased and decaying natural world.

Regarding the issue of whole food supplementation versus isolated vitamin therapy, I shall leave you with these words by food researcher Annemarie Colbin, founder of New York's renowned Natural Gourmet Cookery School for Food and Health:

Nature—our nature—abhors an imbalance…Fragmentation affects foods not only on the cellular, but also on the chemical level. When wheat is refined into white flour, for example, not only does it lose its bran and germ, but some twenty nutrients are also lost or greatly reduced. Enriching the flour—which entails returning four of those twenty nutrients—does not solve the problem. Not only are the added nutrients fewer in number than those present in the original whole wheat; they also lack the **energy** they had when they were simply part of a living, growing plant. It's like cutting off your arm and then fitting you with a prosthetic one—it may have the same form and fulfill some of the same functions, but it is hardly as good as the original. Isolating the components of a living organism and then remixing them will not recreate the living organism.

The logic, to me, seems obvious: *Added nutrients do not contribute to a live energy field.*

In the ecosystem, the living creatures that comprise it are designed to subsist by consuming what the environment provides…Whole foods are simply fresh, natural, edible things, as close to their natural state as possible.[240]

240 Colbin, Annemarie, *Food & Healing*, Ballantine Books, NY, 1996, pages 36-38

RESOURCES

WHOLE FOOD CONCENTRATE SUPPLEMENTS

NutriPlex Formulas, Inc.
P.O. Box 17482
Boulder, CO 80308
—the only recommended whole food supplements
www.nutriplexformulas.com
1-888-595-4752

EDUCATION

Radiant Aliveness
Charles Cropley, N.D.
Education & Seminars for Practitioners
Nutrition & Self-Reliant Healthcare
Videotapes, Books, Training Programs
Boulder, Colorado
www.radiantaliveness.com
1-720-406-9100

Clinical Nutrition Course: Whole Nutrition
University of Natural Medicine
Santa Fe, New Mexico
www.unaturalmedicine.com
1-505-424-7800

BOOKS

Nutritional Insights 1
300 page manual of clinical nutrition, disease etiology &
whole food supplementation for practitioners
Creative Bureau, Inc.
P.O. Box 17231
Boulder, CO 80308

Food & Healing
AnneMarie Colbin
Ballantine Books

The Green Pharmacy
James Duke, Ph.D.
Rodale Press

Herbal Secrets of the Rainforest
Leslie Taylor, N.D.
Prima Health Publishers

Staying Healthy Shopper's Guide
Elson M. Haas, M.D.
Celestial Arts Publishing

CONCLUSIONS

Whole foods, like all other living entities on this planet, are complex and cannot be duplicated by science. The extraction and isolation of one or several substances called "vitamins" cannot serve the biochemical requirements of human beings because such isolated substances lack the synergists and cofactors needed for myriad biochemical functions. Vitamins are dead, lifeless substances when isolated in supplement form. Vitamins by themselves are chemicals; in the original food complex, they are nutrients. To paraphrase my mentor, biochemist and physician Richard P. Murray, D.C., "To feed a person an isolated supplement for the treatment of disease is like giving a person a steering wheel and telling them to drive to the market."

Human beings require whole foods as found in nature, with all of the important and life-supporting constituents intact. When supplementation is needed for severe deficiencies or poor diets, the next best thing to whole, pure, fresh foods are whole food concentrate supplements, not vitamins pills or so-called multivitamins.

About the Author

Vic Shayne, Ph.D., graduate of the University of Florida and the University of Natural Medicine, is a clinical nutritionist, doctor-consultant, whole food supplement formulator and food science researcher. Dr. Shayne is also certified in Chinese Lymphatic Massage and is a practitioner of Chinese Qi Gong Therapy; and is the former director of the Holistic Health & Counseling Center, Carefree, Arizona. Dr. Shayne has written several books, practitioner-newsletters and newspaper articles over the past 21 years on subjects ranging from disease causation to whole food supplementation for health and wellness and in the clinical setting. He is also the editor of ROOTS newsletter for Natural Healthcare Practitioners, Clinical Chiropractic newsletter and HealthxFiles Newsletter. Dr. Shayne is a researcher for, and contributor to the NutriPlex Formulas' Supplement Review and Nutrient Values of Selected Foods.

Dr. Shayne, who practices what he teaches, is an advocate not only of real food nutrition and whole food supplementation, but also an ecology-minded approach to life, with respect to recycling, support of environmental-friendly corporate responsibility, organic farming, alternative fuel usage, elimination of food chemicals and the discontinuation of all pollutants and toxins that endanger our fragile environment. Dr. Shayne also supports the world's forests, rainforests, waterways, oceans and open spaces for the sake of generations to come. He has frequently stated, "The greatest innovations are those which not only benefit and uplift human-kind, but concomitantly preserve Nature, promote peace and contribute to the enrichment of this single planet we all must share."

BIBLIOGRAPHY

Acres, USA, "The Fluoride Menace," March 2000

Airola, Ph.D., N.D., Paavo, *How to Get Well*, Health Plus Publishers, Sherwood, Oregon, 1974, p. 271.

American Society for Nutritional Sciences: Leklem, J.E. (1990) Vitamin B6. In: *Handbook of Vitamins* (I.J. Machlin, ed.), 2nd ed. pp. 341-392. Marcel Dekker, New York, N.Y. and Raiten, D.J. ed. (1995) *Vitamin B6 Metabolism in Pregnancy, Lactation, and Infancy*. CRC Press, Boca Raton, FL.

American Society for Nutritional Sciences 1999

American Society for Nutritional Sciences: Britton, G. (1995) *Structure and properties of carotenoids in relation to function. FASEB J.* 9: 1551-1558 ; and Krinsky, N.I. (1993) *Actions of carotenoids in biological systems. Ann. Rev. Nutr.* 13: 561-587

American Journal of Clinical Nutrition, 1999; 69; 564-571

American Journal of Clinical Nutrition 1999;70:412-419

American Journal of Clinical Nutrition 1999;69:890-897.

American Journal of Public Health 1999;89:322-329

Archives of General Psychiatry, 1999, ;56: 407-412.

Annals of Internal Medicine: Online report 1999. "The Antioxidant Vitamins and Cardiovascular Disease

Armstrong, Ph.D., Thomas, *The Myth of the A.D.D. Child*, Penguin Books, 1995.

Ballantine, M.D., Rudolph, *Diet & Nutrition, A Holistic Approach,* 1978. Himalyan International Institute, Homesdale, PA.

Berkow, M.D., Robert, Editor, *The Merck Manual,* 16th Ed.,, NJ, 1992, page 966.

British Medical Journal 1998;317:1341-45

Braverman, M.D., Eric R. and Carl C. Pfeiffer, M.D., Ph.D., *The Healing Nutrients Within, Facts, findings and New Research on Amino Acids,* Keats Publishing, New Canaan, Connecticut, 1987

Circulation 1998;98:2390-95

Clarkson, Ph.D.,Priscilla M., "Antioxidants: What are They and What Role Do They Play in Physical Activity and Health? " (Abstract from NIH Workshop:The Role of Dietary Supplements for Physically Active People), HealthWorld Online, March, 2000

Colbin, Annemarie, *Food & Healing,* Ballentine Books, NY, 1996, pages 36-38.

Dorlands Illustrated Medical Dictionary, 26th Edition, W.B. Saunders, Philadelphia,1985

Duke, Ph.D. James, "Synergy," *Nature's Herbs Newsletter,* 1999

Duke, Ph.D., James, *The Green Pharmacy,* Rodale Press, Pennsylvania, 1997

Epidemiology 1999;10:49-53

Faelten, Sharon, Ed., *The Complete Book of Vitamins and Minerals,* Rodale Press, Inc., New Jersey, 1988

Fallon, MA, Sally and Mary Enig, Ph.D., *The Ploy of Soy: A Debate on Modern Soy Products,* Price Pottenger Nutrition Foundation, Health Freedom News, September 1995

Fallon, MA, Sally and Mary Enig, Ph.D., "Why Butter is Better," The Price-Pottenger Nutrition Foundation, 1999, Reprinted from *Health Freedom News,* November/December, 1995

Finnegan, John, *The Facts About Fats*, Celestial Arts, Berkeley, CA 1993

Gallagher, Christopher J., "The Role of Vitamin D in the pathogenesis and treatment of osteoporosis." *Journal: J Rheumatol* 1996; (suppl 45)23:15-8

Garrison, MA, R.Ph., Robert and Elizabeth Somer, MA, RD, *The Nutrition Desk Reference*, Keats Publishing, CT, 1995

Golan, Dr. Ralph, *Finding Options for Easing Osteoarthritis*, OnHealth Network Company online; December 02, 1999

Goldberg, I., American Academy of Nutritional Sciences;, ed. (1994) In: *Functional Foods. Designer Foods, Pharmafoods, Nutraceuticals.* Chapman & Hall, New York, NY ; and Moon, T.E. & Micozzi, M.S., eds. (1989) *Nutrition and Cancer Prevention. Investigating the Role of Micronutrients.* Marcel Dekker, Inc., New York, NY

Guyton, M.D., Arthur C., *Function of the Human Body*, W. B. Saunders Company, Philadelphia, 1974

Haas, M.D., Elson, *Staying Healthy With Nutrition*, Celestial Publishing, 1999

Hamilton, Eva May Nunnelley, Eleanor Noss Whitney, Frances Sienkiewicz Sizer, *Nutrition: Concepts and Controversies* West Publishing Company, St. Paul, MN, 1991

Hark, Ph.D., R.D., Lisa, "Vitamin C: Its Role in Health and Prevention

Healthynet/dentistry online: Preventive Dental Health Assn: "The Dangers of Fluoridation & Alternatives to Fluoride; Elke Babluk— Fluoride: Protected Pollutant or Panacea?, 1999; *Scholarly Journal of the International Society for Fluoride Research*, on the web: www.fluoride-journal.com; Val Verlerian, Fluorides & Fluoridation, Leading Edge Research Group, on the web: trufax.or/fluoride/fluorides.html, 1999; Schacter, M.D., Michael, "The Dangers of Fluoride & Fluoridation, on the web at www.healthy.net, 1999; Taylou, DDS,

Joyal, "Fluoride: Dentistry's Boondoggle, on the web at healthynet/dentistry, 2000

Herbert, M.D. Victor., American Society of Nutritional Sciences: (1996) Vitamin B-12. In: *Present Knowledge in Nutrition* (Filer, L.J. & Ziegler, E., eds.), 7th ed., pp. 191-205. International Life Sciences Institute Press, Washington, DC ; and Allen, L.H. & Casterline, J. (1994) Vitamin B-12 deficiency in the elderly: diagnosis and requirements. *Am. J. Clin. Nutr.* 60: 12-14

Hole, John Jr., *Human Anatomy & Physiology*, William C. Brown Company Publishers, Iowa, 1978, page 471.

Hunter, Beatrice Trum, "Food Health Claims: Fact vs. Fiction," *Consumers' Research*, Washington, DC, May 1991, pp. 10-14

Hutchens, Alma R., *Indian Herbology of North America*, Shambhala, Boston, 1991, page 293

International Journal of Cancer 1998;78:430-6

Jha, MD, Prabhat et.al. *Annals of Internal Medicine*: Online report 1999. "The Antioxidant Vitamins and Cardiovascular Disease: A Critical Review of Epidemiologic and Clinical Trial Data" *and* Prabhat Jha, MD, DPhil; Marcus Flather, MBBS, MRCP; Eva Lonn, MD, FRCPC; Michael Farkouh, MD, FRCPC; and Salim Yusuf, DPhil, FRCP: A Critical Review of Epidemiologic and Clinical Trial Data"

Journal of Chromatographic Science, Vol 30, Nov 1992, pages 433-437 : "Natural food-Fruit Vitamin Content," The Natural Food Hub, 1999

Journal of the American College of Cardiology 1996: 28

Journal of the American Geriatrics Society 1998;46:1407-10

*Journal of the American Dietetic Asso*ciation1995;95:493

Journal of the National Cancer Institute 1996; 88

Journal of the National Cancer Institute, 1999; 91:7-8; 60-66.

Journal of the National Cancer Institute 1999;91:605-613

Kava, Ph.D., R.D., Ruth, *Vitamins & Minerals, Does the Epidemiologic Evidence Justify General Supplementation?*, 2nd Ed., American Council on Science and Health, Inc., February 2000

King, Ph.D., Michael W., Department of Medical Biochemistry, Terre Haute Center for Medical Education, Indiana State University, November 1999

King, Ph.D, Michael W., Terre Haute Center for Medical Education, Indiana State University Department of Biochemistry, November 1999 *Food Safety Notebook*, April 1996

Leigh, Evelyn, Herb Reseaerch Foundation, "Soy protein reduces hot flashes,"*Herbs for Health*, September/October 1998

Lindeberg, Staffan, "Cereal Grains," Paleolithic Diet Symposium; Jun 1997

Lininger, Jr., DC, Schuyler, and Alan R. Gaby, MD, et.al., *The Natural Pharmacy*, Healthnotes, Inc., 1999

McBride, Judy, *Agricultural Research/*, November 1996, ARS; Jean Mayer USDA Human Nutrition Research Center on Aging, Tufts University, Boston, MA

McCarrison, M.D., Robert, *Studies in Deficiency Disease,* Henry Frowde and Hodder & Stoughton, London, 1921.

Mills JL; Simpson JL; Cunningham GC; Conley MR; Rhoads GG. Vitamin A and birth defects. *Am J Obstet Gynecol,* 1997 Jul, 177:1, 31-6

Mirkin, M.D., Gabe, citing: Levine, Mark. Proceedings of the National Academy of Sciences. Report #6787 April, 1996

Murray, ND, Michael T., and Jade Beutler, RRT, RCP, *Understanding Fats & Oils,* Progressive Publishing, Encinitas, CA, 1996

Mosby Medical Encylopedia, Signet, Missouri, 1996

National Academy of Sciences, 1989, *Diet & Health, Implications for Reducing Chronic Disease Risk,* National Research Council

Natural Food Hub online: "*Hormone regulatory effect in women*", Natural food-Grains Beans and Seeds, The Natural Food Hub, 2000 UHIS

Natural Food Hub online, The: "Natural food-Fruit Vitamin C Content"

New England Journal of Medicine, Volume 334, No 18.

Olson, J.A. (1994) *Vitamin A, retinoids, and carotenoids. In: Modern Nutrition in Health and Disease* (Shils, M.E., Olson, J.A. & Shike, M., eds), 8th ed., pp. 287-307, Lea & Febiger, Philadelphia, PA

Preventive Medicine 1999;28:333-339

Prior, Ph.D., Ronald L and Cao, Dr. Guohua, *USDA Human Nutrition Research Center on Aging at Tufts, Boston, MA; USDA Agricultural Research Service, July 1997*

Prior, Ph.D., Ronald L., "Bioavailability and Health Benefits of Phytochemicals in Fruits and Vegetables," Phytochemical Research Laboratory, 1999.

Rath, M.D., Mattthias; 1999 *The Doctors' Medical Library*

Raven, Peter H., Director, Missouri Botanical Garden; Engelmann Professor of Botany, Washington University, St. Louis, Missouri and George B Johnson, Professor of Biology, Washington University, St. Louis, Missouri : *Biology,* Third Edition Mosby-Year Book, Inc., Missouri, 1992

Reavley, Nicola, *Vitamins, Etc.* and *Vitamin Update,* Bookman Press, Melbourne, Australia, 1999.

Reavley, Nicola, *The New Encyclopedia of Vitamins, Minerals, Supplements & Herbs*M. Evans & Company, New York, 1999

Reilly, ND, Paul, Clinical Application: Medicago sativa extracts, Volume 1, Number 1, 1999

Reuben, C.A., Carolyn and Joan Priestley, M.D., *Essential Supplements for Women*, Perigee Books, New York, 1988

Romero, M.A,. Rodriguez, *et al* 'Determination of Vitamin C and Organic acids in various fruits by HPLC'

Ronzio, Ph.D., Robert, *The Encyclopedia of Nutrition and Good Health*, Facts on File, Inc., New York, 1997

Sackheim, George and Ronald M. Schultz, *Chemistry for the Health Sciences*, The Macmillan Company, New York, 1973

Schardt, David, "Phytoestrogens for Menopause," *Nutrition Action Health Letter*, January/February 2000, Volume 27, Number 1, Center for Science in the Public Interest

Seibold, MS, Ronald L., *Cereal Grass, What's in it for you!*, Wilderness Community Education Foundation, Kansas, 1990, pages 24-25

Shayne, Ph.D., Vic, ed. *Nutritional Insights I*, Creative Bureau, Inc., Boulder, CO, 1998.

Smolin & Grosvenor, *Nutrition, Science & Applications*, Saunders College Publishing, 1994.

Sporn, M.B., Roberts, A.B. & Goodman, D.S. (eds.) (1994) *The Retinoids*, 2nd ed. Raven Press, New York, NY.

Sterling, M.A., M.N.I.M.H., Keith, Medicinal Plants, Volume 15, Issue 1, January 1992.

Tanphaichitr, V., American Society of Nutritional Sciences: (1994) *Thiamin. In: Modern Nutrition in Health and Disease* (Shils, M.E., Olson, J.A., & Shike, M., eds.), 8th ed., vol. 1, pp. 359-365. Lea & Febiger, Philadelphia, PA, and Tan, G.H., Farnell, G.F., Hensrud, D.D. & Litin, S.C. (1994) Acute Wernicke's encephalopathy attributable to pure dietary thiamine deficiency. *Mayo. Clin. Proc.* 69: 849-850.

Thibodeau, Gary A., *Anthony's Textbook of Anatomy and Physiology* 13th Edition, Times Mirror/Mosby College Publishing, St. Louis, MO

"Vitamin E from Foods May Reduce Women's Heart Disease Risk,"
HealthNews from the publishers of the *New England Journal of Medicine,*
June 4, 1996; OnHealth, 2000 OnHealth Network Company

Vitamin News, July 1996

Vitamin News for October 1999

Vitamin Update, Bookman Press online, 1998

Vitamin Update, July 1996

Vitamin News, April /May 1997

Vitamin News for April/May 1997

Wootan, Dr. Margo, "Trans Fat Spells Double Trouble for Arteries, *What the Food Labels Don't Tell You," Nutrition Action Healthletter,* Center for Science in the Public Interest, 1996

INDEX

Breinigsville, PA USA
20 March 2011
257982BV00001B/85/A